BMA

Ophthalmology at a Glance

Ophthalmology at a Glance

Jane Olver

BSc(Hons), MB BS, DO, FRCS, FRCOphth
Consultant Ophthalmic, Oculoplastic and Orbital Surgeon
Western Eye and Charing Cross Hospitals
Imperial College Healthcare NHS Trust;
Director Clinica London
London, UK

Lorraine Cassidy

MB, DO, FRCSI, FRCOphth
Professor of Ophthalmology
Trinity College, Dublin;
Consultant Ophthalmologist, Neuro-ophthalmologist and Oculoplastic Surgeon
The Royal Victoria Eye and Ear Hospital;
The Adelaide and Meath Hospital, incorporating the National Childrens' Hospital
Dublin, Ireland

Gurjeet Jutley

BM, BSc(Hons)
Specialist Registrar
Moorfields Eye Hospital
London, UK

Laura Crawley

BSc(Hons), MB, ChB(Hons), MRCP, FRCOphth
Glaucoma Fellow
Imperial College Healthcare NHS Trust
London, UK

Second Edition

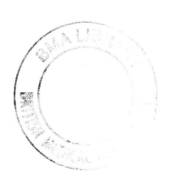

WILEY Blackwell

This edition first published 2014 © Jane Olver, Lorraine Cassidy, Gurjeet Jutley and Laura Crawley
First edition published 2005 by Blackwell Science Ltd

Registered Office
John Wiley & Sons Ltd, The Atrium, Southern Gate, Chichester, West Sussex, PO19 8SQ, UK

Editorial Offices
350 Main Street, Malden, MA 02148-5020, USA
9600 Garsington Road, Oxford, OX4 2DQ, UK
The Atrium, Southern Gate, Chichester, West Sussex, PO19 8SQ, UK

For details of our global editorial offices, for customer services, and for information about how to apply for permission to reuse the copyright material in this book please see our website at www.wiley.com/wiley-blackwell.

The right of Jane Olver, Lorraine Cassidy, Gurjeet Jutley and Laura Crawley to be identified as the authors of this work has been asserted in accordance with the UK Copyright, Designs and Patents Act 1988.

Wiley also publishes its books in a variety of electronic formats. Some content that appears in print may not be available in electronic books.

Designations used by companies to distinguish their products are often claimed as trademarks. All brand names and product names used in this book are trade names, service marks, trademarks or registered trademarks of their respective owners. The publisher is not associated with any product or vendor mentioned in this book.

Limit of Liability/Disclaimer of Warranty: While the publisher and author(s) have used their best efforts in preparing this book, they make no representations or warranties with respect to the accuracy or completeness of the contents of this book and specifically disclaim any implied warranties of merchantability or fitness for a particular purpose. It is sold on the understanding that the publisher is not engaged in rendering professional services and neither the publisher nor the author shall be liable for damages arising herefrom. If professional advice or other expert assistance is required, the services of a competent professional should be sought.

Library of Congress Cataloging-in-Publication Data

Olver, Jane, author.
  Ophthalmology at a glance / Jane Olver, Lorraine Cassidy, Gurjeet Jutley, Laura Crawley.—Second edition.
       p. ; cm.—(At a glance)
  Includes bibliographical references and index.
    ISBN 978-1-4051-8473-1 (paper)
  I. Cassidy, Lorraine, author.   II. Crawley, Laura, active 2014, author.   III. Jutley, Gurjeet, author.
IV. Title.   V. Series: At a glance series (Oxford, England)
  [DNLM: 1. Eye Diseases–Examination Questions.   2. Ophthalmology–methods–Examination Questions.   WW   18.2]
  RE50
  617.7–dc23
                                        2013038050

A catalogue record for this book is available from the British Library.

Cover image: Courtesy of Jane Olver, Lorraine Cassidy, Gurjeet Jutley and Laura Crawley
Cover design by Meaden Creative

Set in 9/11.5 pt Times by Toppan Best-set Premedia Limited
Printed and bound in Malaysia by Vivar Printing Sdn Bhd

2   2015

Contents

Preface to the second edition

Ophthalmology at a Glance is aimed at the medical student, specialist trainee or general practitioner. It is a great pleasure to write the second edition of Ophthalmology at a Glance and introduce the reader to the many advances that have occurred in ophthalmology since 2004, not least with the training syllabus, corneal refractive surgery and cataract surgery, and in the treatment of medical retinal disorders. We hope that you find all of these advances reflected in this new edition.

We aim to provide the fundamentals of ophthalmology, starting with the basics of how to take a history, how to correct refractive errors, do the eye examination, the management of acute eye problems, and causes of gradual loss of vision in Parts 1 to 5. We will then discuss the areas of the eye and visual disturbance in more detail in the latter parts 6–13. The largest subspecialty part is vitreo-retinal, which in this edition has been expanded to include chapters on tropical ophthalmology by Sophia Pathai.

We have also introduced a new chapter dedicated to ocular oncology by Mandeep Sagoo and Karim Hammamji, an area that medical students, newly-trained doctors and GPs should be aware of. It is exciting in this second edition to have two new co-authors: Gurjeet Jutley, Specialist Trainee, and Laura Crawley, Glaucoma Fellow, who have both worked extremely hard to update many of the chapters, provide new images and write the case studies for the website.

We hope that the reader will find this book helpful for their studies, when seeing patients in clinic and to help increase their interest in ophthalmology.

Jane Olver, London 2014

Preface to first edition

This book is intended primarily for medical students and junior doctors preparing for examinations (regardless of whether they are medical or surgical). In addition, we hope that general practitioners and non-ophthalmic consultants who care for patients with eye diseases will find this book invaluable in its simplicity and clarity. We have tried to create a balanced, up-to-date, practical book. Blackwell's have supported our need for the extensive colour pictures and diagrams which characterize this 'visual' subject.

Ophthalmology at a Glance took form in London around the time that Lorraine Cassidy was about to go to Dublin to become Professor of Ophthalmology. Slowly, we gathered together a team of colleagues and friends who over 2–3 years all pulled together—were cajoled?—into writing this book. As editors, we have knitted together our own and their contributing work. We are incredibly grateful to everyone who made this book a reality.

Jane Olver and Lorraine Cassidy
London and Dublin, 2004

Acknowledgements

Thanks to Ingrid Hurtado, the Clinica London Nurse, for taking many of the pictures for this second edition (with the three authors) at Clinica London on 1 September 2012. We also acknowledge Susan Downes for her contributory photos in Chapters 45 and 46.

A special thank you to Mr Nigel Davies, Consultant Ophthalmic Surgeon Chelsea and Westminster Hospital, and Michel Michaelides, Consultant Ophthalmologist and Clinica Senior Lecturer, Moorfields Eye Hospital and UCL Institute of Ophthalmology, for editing the Medical Retina chapters.

Contributors

Contributors to the second edition

Karim Hammamji, MD, FRCSC, DipABO
Fellow in Ocular Oncology
Moorfields Eye Hospital and St. Bartholomew's Hospital
London, UK

Sophia Pathai, MBBS, BSc(Hons), MRCOphth, MSc, PhD
Clinical Research Fellow
International Centre for Eye Health
London School of Hygiene & Tropical Medicine
London, UK

Mandeep S. Sagoo, MB, PhD, MRCOphth, FRCS(Ed)
Senior Lecturer and Consultant Ophthalmic Surgeon
UCL Institute of Ophthalmology, Moorfields Eye Hospital and St.
Bartholomew's and the Royal London Hospitals
London, UK

With thanks

Nigel Davies, MA, MB, BS, PhD, FRCOphth
Consultant Ophthalmic Surgeon
Chelsea and Westminster Hospital
London, UK

Michel Michaelides, BSc, MB, BS, MD(Res), FRCOphth, FACS
Consultant Ophthalmic Surgeon
Moorfields Eye Hospital;
Clinical Senior Lecturer
UCL Institute of Ophthalmology
London, UK

Contributors to the first edition

Jonathan Barnes, BSc, FRCOphth
Consultant Ophthalmic Surgeon
Luton and Dunstable Hospital
Lewsey Road
Luton, UK

Anne Bolton
Head of Ophthalmic Imaging
Oxford Eye Hospital
Woodstock Road
Oxford, UK

Susan Downes, MD, FRCOphth
Consultant Ophthalmic Surgeon
Oxford Eye Hospital
Woodstock Road
Oxford, UK

Veronica Ferguson, FRCS, FRCOphth
Consultant Ophthalmic Surgeon
Charing Cross Hospital
London, UK

Sanjay Gautama, MB, BS
Consultant Anaesthetist
St Mary's Hospital NHS Trust
London, UK

Anthony Kwan
Vitreoretinal Fellow
Moorfields Eye Hospital
London, UK

Jane Leach, FRCOphth
Consultant Ophthalmologist
The Royal Victoria Eye & Ear Hospital
Dublin, Ireland

Damien Louis
Staff Ophthalmologist
Melbourne, Australia

Raj Maini, FRCOphth
Consultant Ophthalmologist
Department of Ophthalmology
Charing Cross Hospital
London, UK

Raman Malhotra, FRCOphth
Consultant Ophthalmic Surgeon
Corneoplastic Unit
Queen Victoria Hospital
East Grinstead, Sussex, UK

Bernadette McCarry, DBO
Teaching Orthoptist
Moorfields Eye Hospital
London, UK

Suzanne Mitchell, FRCOphth
Consultant Ophthalmic Surgeon
Chelsea and Westminster Hospital
London, UK

Jugnoo Rahi
The Royal Victoria Eye and Ear Hospital
Dublin, Ireland

Dilani Siriwardena, FRCOphth
Consultant Ophthalmic Surgeon
Moorfields Eye Hospital
London, UK

Ursula Vogt, MD
Director
Contact Lens Department
Western Eye Hospital
London, UK

How to use your textbook

Features contained within your textbook

Each topic is presented in a double-page spread with clear, easy-to-follow diagrams supported by succinct explanatory text.

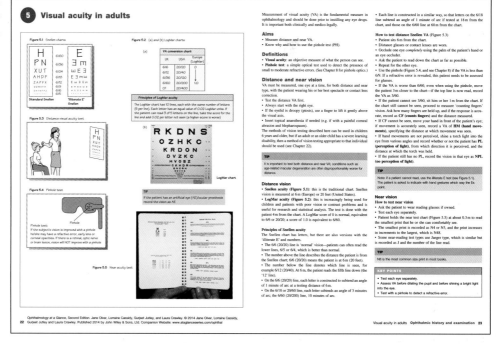

Key point boxes summarize the need-to-know information.
Further reading boxes show how to find out more online or in your library.

Tip boxes give further insight into topics.
Warning boxes highlight important cautionary points.

The anytime, anywhere textbook

Wiley E-Text

Your book is also available to purchase as a **Wiley E-Text: Powered by VitalSource** version—a digital, interactive version of this book which you own as soon as you download it.

Your **Wiley E-Text** allows you to:

Search: Save time by finding terms and topics instantly in your book, your notes, even your whole library (once you've downloaded more textbooks)

Note and highlight: Colour code, highlight and make digital notes right in the text so you can find them quickly and easily

Organize: Keep books, notes and class materials organized in folders inside the application

Share: Exchange notes and highlights with friends, classmates and study groups

Upgrade: Your textbook can be transferred when you need to change or upgrade computers

Link: Link directly from the page of your interactive textbook to all of the material contained on the companion website

The **Wiley E-Text** version will also allow you to copy and paste any photograph or illustration into assignments, presentations and your own notes.

To access your Wiley E-Text:

• Visit   www.vitalsource.com/software/bookshelf/downloads   to download the Bookshelf application to your computer, laptop, tablet or mobile device.

• Open the Bookshelf application on your computer and register for an account.

• Follow the registration process.

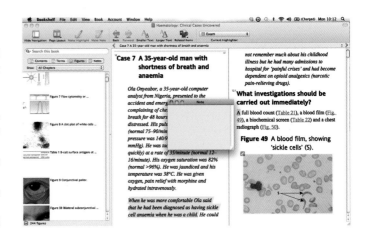

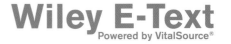

The VitalSource Bookshelf can now be used to view your Wiley E-Text on iOS, Android and Kindle Fire!

- **For iOS:** Visit the app store to download the VitalSource Bookshelf: **http://bit.ly/17ib3XS**
- **For Android:** Visit the Google Play Market to download the VitalSource Bookshelf: **http://bit.ly/ ZMEGvo**
- **For Kindle Fire, Kindle Fire 2 or Kindle Fire HD:** Simply install the VitalSource Bookshelf onto your Fire (see how at **http://bit.ly/11BVFn9**). You can now sign in with the email address and password you used when you created your VitalSource Bookshelf Account.

Full E-Text support for mobile devices is available at: **http://support.vitalsource.com**

CourseSmart

CourseSmart gives you instant access (via computer or mobile device) to this Wiley-Blackwell e-book and its extra electronic functionality, at 40% off the recommended retail print price. See all the benefits at: **www.coursesmart.com/students**

Instructors . . . receive your own digital desk copies!

CourseSmart also offers instructors an immediate, efficient, and environmentally-friendly way to review this book for your course.

For more information visit **www.coursesmart.com/instructors**.

With CourseSmart, you can create lecture notes quickly with copy and paste, and share pages and notes with your students. Access your **CourseSmart** digital book from your computer or mobile device instantly for evaluation, class preparation, and as a teaching tool in the classroom.

Simply sign in at **http://instructors.coursesmart.com/bookshelf** to download your Bookshelf and get started. To request your desk copy, hit 'Request Online Copy' on your search results or book product page.

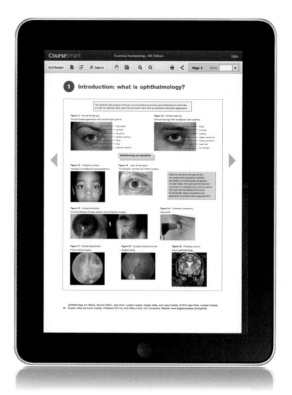

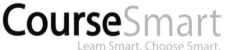

We hope you enjoy using your new book. Good luck with your studies!

About the companion website

Don't forget to visit the companion website for this book:

 www.ataglanceseries.com/ophthal

There you will find valuable material designed to enhance your learning, including:
• Case studies to test your knowledge
• All photos from the book in PowerPoint format
• Interactive flashcards for self-test

1 Introduction: what is ophthalmology?

The medicine and surgery of the eye, its surrounding structures and connections to the brain, in order to maintain clear, pain-free and useful vision with an aesthetic attractive appearance

Figure 1.1 Normal female eye
Normal female appearance with arched high eyebrow

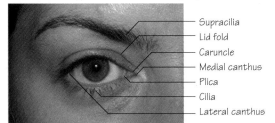

- Supracilia
- Lid fold
- Caruncle
- Medial canthus
- Plica
- Cilia
- Lateral canthus

Figure 1.2 Normal male eye
Normal male eye with straighter lower eyebrow

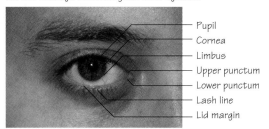

- Pupil
- Cornea
- Limbus
- Upper punctum
- Lower punctum
- Lash line
- Lid margin

Ophthalmology sub-specialties

Figure 1.3 Paediatric ptosis:
managed in strabismus and paediatrics

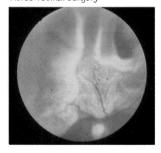

Figure 1.4 Lower lid entropion
Oculoplastic, lacrimal and orbital surgery

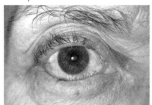

Vision is central to the way we live; our social world, education, mobility and ability to communicate all depend on clear vision. The eyes and the face are important for interpersonal communication – 'the eyes are the window of the soul'. Economically, many occupations are dependent on precise visual requirements

Figure 1.5 Corneal laceration
External disease: Cornea, catarct and refractive surgery

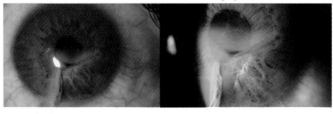

Figure 1.6 Goldmann tonometry
Glaucoma

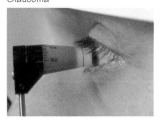

Figure 1.7 Retinal detachment
Vitreo-retinal surgery

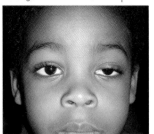

Figure 1.8 Occluded retinal arteriole
Medical retina

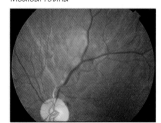

Figure 1.9 Pituitary tumour
Neuro-ophthalmology

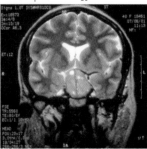

Ophthalmology at a Glance, Second Edition. Jane Olver, Lorraine Cassidy, Gurjeet Jutley, and Laura Crawley. © 2014 Jane Olver, Lorraine Cassidy, Gurjeet Jutley and Laura Crawley. Published 2014 by John Wiley & Sons, Ltd. Companion Website: www.ataglanceseries.com/ophthal

What is ophthalmology?

Ophthalmology is a large subject for a very small organ: it is the medical and surgical care of the eye (Figures 1.1 and 1.2), the adjacent adnexal and periocular area and the visual system. It encompasses the upper and mid-face, eyebrows and eyelids, lacrimal system and orbit, as well as the globe and eye muscles, optic nerve and nervous connections all the way back to the visual cortex. Many medical conditions have ocular features as their first presentation, for example in diabetes, cardiovascular disease, rheumatology, neurology, endocrinology and oncology. There are strong links and overlap with maxillofacial, plastic, otolaryngological, dermatology and neurosurgery. There are links with neuroradiology and pathology. Ophthalmology combines medical and surgical skills and uses minimally invasive microsurgery and lasers as well as delicate plastic surgical techniques.

Type of patients

Predominantly the very young and the elderly. Also, middle-aged patients with thyroid eye disease, diabetes or inherited disorders. Ophthalmic trauma affects particularly the young adult. Very few eye patients become ill and die. Most remain ambulatory and are seen as outpatients or have day-case surgery.

Team

General practitioners, eye casualty officers, hospital ophthalmologists, medical physicists, optometrists, orthoptists and ophthalmic nurse practitioners all collaborate in the investigation and management of ophthalmic patients.

Sub-specialties

The eye can be subdivided into several sub-specialty areas. Some ophthalmologists practice general ophthalmology alone, although most have a significant sub-specialty interest. Sub-specialties include:
• Paediatric and strabismus (Figure 1.3)
• Oculoplastic, lacrimal and orbital (including oncology) (Figure 1.4)
• External eye disease, including contact lenses
• Cornea and refractive surgery, and cataracts (Figure 1.5)
• Glaucoma (Figure 1.6)
• Vitreo-retinal surgery (Figure 1.7)
• Medical retina (Figure 1.8)
• Neuro-ophthalmology (Figure 1.9)
• Tropical ophthalmology.

Ophthalmology at medical school

Exposure to ophthalmology at the undergraduate level is rather limited, and the onus is on the student to make the most of every opportunity. One should read this book prior to the attachment and use it to further reference conditions seen in clinic. Taking structured histories and becoming accustomed with using the slit lamp and direct ophthalmoscopy are the aims of the attachment. Students with keen interest can choose to do a specialist study module in ophthalmology: students with a keen interest can choose to do a specialty module in ophthalmology where they can observe, theatre, administering botulinum toxin and laser therapy and attend multi-disciplinary team meetings with the other specialties.

How to get into ophthalmology

Firstly, one must be certain that one possesses the skills to become a good ophthalmologist. Use the cataract simulator (available at the Royal College of Ophthalmologists and Moorfields Eye Hospitals) to experience the intricacies of intraocular surgery and ensure you have the hand–eye coordination to excel at this difficult skill. Ophthalmology is an exquisitely competitive specialty, and one must ensure optimal preparation prior to selection processes. In order to get short-listed for interviews, showing commitment is key. Undertake the microsurgical skills course at the Royal College to ensure you are able to start surgery at specialist trainee one (ST1) level. Organize a 2-week 'taster' programme during your foundation training, which will also afford you insight as to the daily routine of ophthalmology training. Participate in an audit project in your local trust: if you can complete the cycle and implement change to the service, this will provide the basis to present your work at meetings. Attend the local and regional teaching programme at your deanery; if you are able to present any ophthalmic cases you have seen, all the better. Although it is not compulsory, you may wish to prepare for and sit the part one Fellowship of the Royal College of Ophthalmologists (FRCOphth) examination (no clinical experience is required to take this predominantly basic science and physics examination).

Once short-listed, the interviews are a difficult step, testing a range of skills and the ability to remain composed in an unfamiliar situation. Critical appraisal, situation judgment, role-play and manual dexterity are all tested in a 90-minute marathon!

Ophthalmology is currently a run-through specialty from the ST1 level. Targets are set throughout regular intervals and include:
• Completing the part one FRCOphth examination and 50 cataract extractions by the end of ST2.
• Passing the refraction certificate by ST4.
• Completing the exit exam and 300 cataract extractions by the advanced subspecialist training year.

Colleges
• Royal College of Ophthalmologists: www.rcophth.ac.uk
• Royal College of Surgeons of Edinburgh: www.rcsed.ac.uk
• Irish College of Ophthalmologists: www.seeico.com

Education website
• Success in MRCOphth: http://www.mrcophth.com

Eye associations
• American Academy Ophthalmology: www.aao.org
• American Associated Ophthalmic Plastic and Reconstructive Surgery: www.asoprs.org
• American Association Paediatric Ophthalmology and Strabismus: www.aapos.org
• Association for Research Vision and Ophthalmology: www.arvo.org
• British Oculoplastic Surgery Society: www.bopss.org

FURTHER READING

1 *The Wills Eye Manual. Office and Emergency Room Diagnosis and Treatment of Eye Disease.* Douglas J. Rhee and Mark F. Pyfer.
2 *Clinical Anatomy of the Eye.* Richard S. Snell and Micheal A. Lemp.
3 *Ophthalmology. An Illustrated Text.* M. Batterbury and B. Bowling.
4 *Training in Ophthalmology: The Essential Clinical Curriculum.* V Sundaram, A Barsam, A Alwitry and PT Khaw.

KEY POINTS
• Ophthalmology is multidisciplinary.
• Interfaces with medicine.
• Involves microsurgery.

2 Medical student aims

Essential ophthalmic skills

Figure 2.1 Measure visual acuity

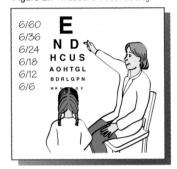

Figure 2.2 Detect an abnormal pupil

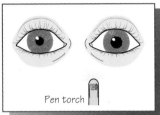

Pen torch

Figure 2.3 Detect a squint

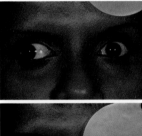

Figure 2.4 (a) Examine the red reflex and (b) use an ophthalmoscope
(a)

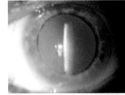

(b)

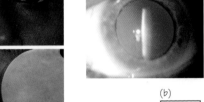

Figure 2.5 Perform a confrontational visual field test

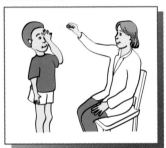

Figure 2.6 Examine the fundus

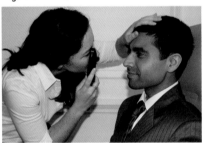

Figure 2.7 Identify a normal disc

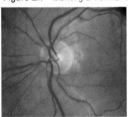

Figure 2.8 Identify (a) diabetic retinopathy and (b) hypertensive retinopathy

(a)

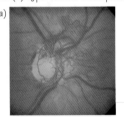

(b)

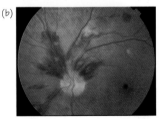

Figure 2.9 Identify (a) glaucomatous cupping and (b) papilloedema

(a)

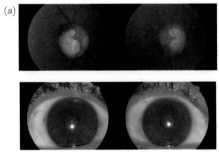

(b)

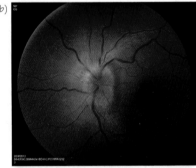

Figure 2.10 Recognize common ophthalmic conditions, *e.g.* Meibomian cyst (chalazion)

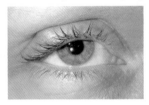

Figure 2.11 *Recognize ophthalmic emergencies, e.g. acute angle-closure glaucoma*

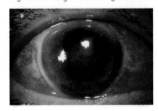

Ophthalmology at a Glance, Second Edition. Jane Olver, Lorraine Cassidy, Gurjeet Jutley, and Laura Crawley. © 2014 Jane Olver, Lorraine Cassidy, Gurjeet Jutley and Laura Crawley. Published 2014 by John Wiley & Sons, Ltd. Companion Website: www.ataglanceseries.com/ophthal

Systematic approach

The time spent in ophthalmology at the undergraduate level is very short, so a systematic approach is needed in order to ensure that the necessary skills and topics are met. Try to cover the items identified in this chapter and refer back to it as a checklist. Many students arrive at our clinics feeling daunted and underprepared due to a lack of experience and knowledge in the field. We advise them to think of it as any other specialty: understand the anatomy, the basic physiology and the pathology. Further to that, it will be our job in clinic to introduce you to unfamiliar equipment, such as the indirect ophthalmoscope, Goldman's tonometer, exophthalmometer and so on. We will help facilitate the examination and slowly work up your skills in order to reach a diagnosis: do not worry if at first you are unable to visualize and appreciate very little! It gets easier, especially with the help of this book.

Aims

The aim of this book is to provide a balanced understanding of clinical ophthalmology and equip the reader with the knowledge and skills to identify, treat or refer common eye disorders.

Core knowledge

A basic understanding of:
- ocular physiology and pharmacology
- neuro-anatomy
- optics.

Medical student objectives

There are **essential ophthalmic skills** such as taking a history, useful **practical skills** such as putting in eye drops, **things to do when you visit the eye department** such as watch a visual field being done and, lastly, **essential clinical topics** such as the red eye.

Essential ophthalmic skills

- Take an **ophthalmic history**.
- Measure **visual acuity** (Figure 2.1) using Snellen and Logmar charts, with and without a pinhole.
- Detect an abnormal **pupil** (Figure 2.2), such as a fixed dilated pupil, Horner's pupil or afferent pupillary defect using a pen torch.
- Examine the **eye movements** and extraocular muscle function. Detect a **squint** using the cover test (Figure 2.3). Differentiate between a paralytic and non-paralytic squint.
- Examine the **red reflex** (Figure 2.4) and recognize leukocoria.
- Perform a confrontation **visual field test** (Figure 2.5), and detect a bitemporal hemianopia and homonymous hemianopia.
- Use a direct ophthalmoscope to (i) **examine the fundus** (Figure 2.6) **and identify a normal disc** (Figure 2.7); (ii) detect **diabetic retinopathy** (Figure 2.8a) and **hypertensive retinopathy** (Figure 2.8b); and (iii) detect **papilloedema** (Figure 2.9b), glaucomatous **cupping** of the optic nerve head (Figure 2.9a) and a pale disc with **optic atrophy**.
- Recognize common ophthalmic lid conditions (e.g. benign eyelid **chalazion**) (Figure 2.10) and malignant eyelid **basal cell carcinoma**.
- Recognize **ophthalmic emergencies** (e.g. acute angle closure glaucoma) (Figure 2.11) and orbital cellulitis.

Things to do when you visit the eye department

- Attend (i) a general eye or primary eye clinic, and (ii) a specialist eye clinic.
- Attend an eye casualty clinic.
- Observe an orthoptist assessing ocular motility in a child or adult.
- Observe an automated visual field test being done.
- Watch a phaco-cataract extraction operation.
- Watch an eyelid lump being incised or excised, for example incision and curettage (I&C) of a chalazion.
- See retinal laser treatment for diabetic retinopathy.
- Watch an intra-ocular injection for age related macular degeneration.

KEY POINTS

- Visit the eye department and theatre.
- Know essential clinical topics.
- Gain essential practical skills.

3 Social and occupational aspects of vision

Table 3.1 Blindness is a severe form of visual impairment and must be defined. The WHO classification helps:

Category of vision	Level of visual impairment	Visual acuity in better eye with optical correction
Normal vision	Slight if visual acuity <6/7.5 (20/30)	6/18 (20/40) or better
Low vision Low vision	Visual impairment (VI) Severe visual impairment (SVI)	Vision between 6/18 and 6/60 (20/40–20/100) Vision between 6/60 and 3/60 (20/100–20/300)
Blindness	Blind (BL)	Less than 3/60 to no light perception or visual field ≤ 10° around central fixation

Definitions:
BL = Blind
SVI = Severely visually impaired
VI = Visually impaired

Figure 3.1 A visual acuity of 6/12 (20/30) or worse in the better eye **excludes** entry into the following occupations:

Driving including taxi drivers

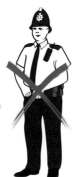

Entry to armed forces

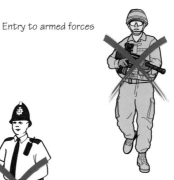

Entry to the police force

Fire brigade

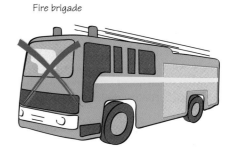

Bus driver

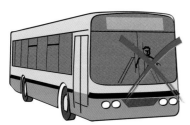

Pilot

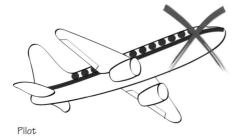

DVLA Visual Standards for Driving for ordinary driving licence

NB Professional and Vocational licence eyesight regulations are stricter for Large Goods Vehicle (LGV) and Passenger Carrying Vehicle (PCV) licences

- Visual acuity: 'read in good light (with the aid of glasses or contact lenses if worn) a registration mark fixed to a motor vehicle and containing letters and figures 79.4 mm high at a distance of 20.5 m'. This is equivalent to between 6/9 (20/25) and 6/12 (20/30)

- Visual fields: 'a field of vision of at least 120° on the horizontal measured by a Goldman perimeter using a III4e target setting (or automated perimetry equivalent), with no defect in binocular field within 20° of fixation above or below fixation, i.e. total 40°'

A patient can have diplopia in extremes of vision and still be allowed to drive. If in doubt, the patient should contact the DVLA

For LGV and PCV a minimum vision of 3/60 unaided, in each eye, is required, as long as it corrects to 6/9 in the better eye and 6/12 in the worst eye – monocular driving or any field defect is a contraindication

DVLA: www.dvla.gov.uk/drivers/medical/vision-recall.htm

Ophthalmology at a Glance, Second Edition. Jane Olver, Lorraine Cassidy, Gurjeet Jutley, and Laura Crawley. © 2014 Jane Olver, Lorraine Cassidy,
18 Gurjeet Jutley and Laura Crawley. Published 2014 by John Wiley & Sons, Ltd. Companion Website: www.ataglanceseries.com/ophthal

Our social and economic lives are dependent on good vision. Refractive errors remain the single most important cause of impaired vision worldwide, and they are an important and easily preventable cause of visual impairment and severe visual impairment in developing countries (Table 3.1). Simply providing good optometry services to a wider world population will go far to meet these needs. Vision 2020 aims to tackle the main causes of blindness. Reducing infective and malnutrition-related causes of blindness will also help.

Aims
• Recognize the differing needs of emerging and developed countries.
• Know the main causes of blindness in children and adults.
• Know the visual requirements for driving.

Some simple facts

Blindness worldwide:
• One adult becomes blind every 5 seconds.
• One child becomes blind every minute.
• Over 45 million adults and 1.5 million children are blind.
• The global cost of blindness (lost work and support) is over US$167 000 million per annum.
  Developing and emerging countries:
• Most blind and severely visually impaired (SVI) people are in developing countries.
• Most of these cases are preventable.
• Limited resources are available for treatment (e.g. cataract surgery).
  Emerging and developed countries:
• Most preventable blinding diseases are eliminated.
• Refractive problems are largely solved by glasses, contact lenses and laser refractive surgery.

United Kingdom and developed industrialized countries
Children
Approximately 1 per 1000 children are visually impaired (VI) or SVI, and they may have associated learning, hearing, speech–language or motility impairment. This can have a profound impact on education, employment and social prospects.

Although many of the causes of blindness in children are untreatable, there is much that can be done to help visual rehabilitation with low-vision aids and specific educational and developmental intervention.

The major causes of childhood visual impairment include:
• visual pathway or cerebral visual impairment
• inherited retinal dystrophies (see Chapter 44)
• congenital cataract, microphthalmia, optic nerve atrophy and optic nerve hypoplasia.
• retinopathy of prematurity.

Adults
The incidence and major causes of partial sight or blindness in the United Kingdom at various ages are given in this table:

Age in years	Incidence per 100 000 per year	Major causes of visual impairment and blindness
16–64	13	Diabetic retinopathy Macular degeneration Hereditary retinal disorders Optic atrophy
65–74	122	Age-related macular degeneration
75–84	471	Glaucoma
85 and over	1038	Cataract

Economic blindness
A visual acuity of worse than 6/12 in the better eye in adults can be considered 'economic blindness' as it:
• precludes driving;
• prevents entry into certain occupations (Figure 3.1);
• decreases ability to function in the workplace;
• increases risk of serious morbidity;
• increases social isolation and the risk of psychological problems, including depression; and
• decreases overall quality of life and is associated with increased (doubling) overall risk of death.

Services and support in the United Kingdom and Ireland (children and adults)
• *National registers of partial sight and blindness.* Certification as partially sighted or blind (approximately equivalent to SVI or BL) is voluntary. It is the main mechanism for ensuring access to statutory economic benefits and relevant social services. It provides national data about levels of visual impairment.
• *Statement of Educational Needs (SEN).* It is a UK legal requirement to assess and regularly review the educational needs of children with SVI in a 'Statement of Educational Needs'. Children registered blind in Ireland are assessed by the visually impaired assessment team (VICAT). The SEN or VICAT report determines the educational placement, support and facilities provided by the government. VI children are educated in mainstream schools with support from an advisory teacher, special visual impairment units integrated within mainstream schools, schools and colleges for the visually impaired or residential schools for children with special needs.

TIP: Certification of partially sighted or blind

• Both visual acuity and visual field are considered.
• A patient can be SVI or BL in one eye and even have a prosthetic eye, but if the other eye sees 6/12 with a good visual field, they cannot be registered partially sighted or blind.

Useful websites

• Action for Blind People: www.afbp.org
• Royal National Institute for the Blind: www.rnib.org.uk
• Sense: www.sense.org.uk
• National Council for the Blind of Ireland: www.ncbi.ie

KEY POINTS

• Diabetic retinopathy is the commonest cause of blindness in the working age group.
• Age-related macular degeneration accounts for over 50% of blind or partially sighted registrations in Western Europe and the United States.
• Both good visual acuity and field of vision are necessary for driving.

Figure 4.1 Standard eye examination record

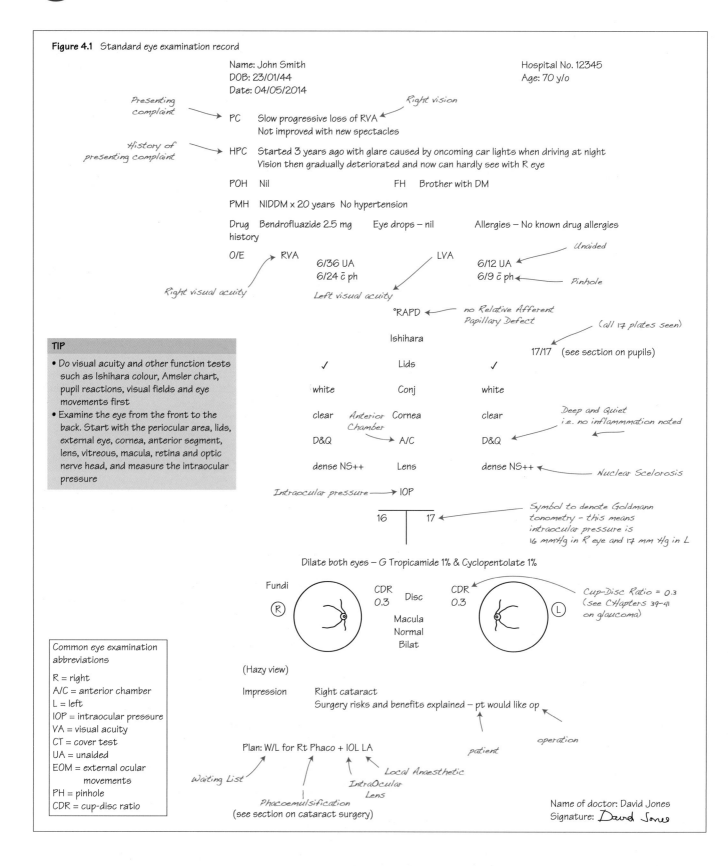

Name: John Smith
DOB: 23/01/44
Date: 04/05/2014

Hospital No. 12345
Age: 70 y/o

Presenting complaint → PC   Slow progressive loss of RVA ← *Right vision*
Not improved with new spectacles

History of presenting complaint → HPC   Started 3 years ago with glare caused by oncoming car lights when driving at night
Vision then gradually deteriorated and now can hardly see with R eye

POH   Nil   FH   Brother with DM

PMH   NIDDM x 20 years No hypertension

Drug history   Bendrofluazide 2.5 mg   Eye drops – nil   Allergies – No known drug allergies

O/E   → RVA   6/36 UA   LVA   6/12 UA   ← *Unaided*
6/24 c̄ ph   6/9 c̄ ph   ← *Pinhole*

Right visual acuity   *Left visual acuity*

°RAPD ← *no Relative Afferent Papillary Defect*

Ishihara   17/17   (see section on pupils)   ← *(all 17 plates seen)*

✓   Lids   ✓

white   Conj   white

clear   *Anterior Chamber* Cornea   clear   *Deep and Quiet i.e. no inflammation noted*

D&Q   → A/C   D&Q ←

dense NS++   Lens   dense NS++ ←   *Nuclear Sclerosis*

Intraocular pressure → IOP

16 | 17 ← *Symbol to denote Goldmann tonometry – this means intraocular pressure is 16 mmHg in R eye and 17 mm Hg in L*

Dilate both eyes – G Tropicamide 1% & Cyclopentolate 1%

Fundi   ⓇR   CDR 0.3   Disc   CDR 0.3   ⓁL   *Cup-Disc Ratio = 0.3 (see Chapters 39–41 on glaucoma)*

Macula Normal Bilat

(Hazy view)

Impression   Right cataract
Surgery risks and benefits explained – pt would like op ← *operation*

patient

Plan: W/L for Rt Phaco + IOL LA

Waiting List   *Phacoemulsification (see section on cataract surgery)*   *IntraOcular Lens*   *Local Anaesthetic*

Name of doctor: David Jones
Signature: *David Jones*

TIP
- Do visual acuity and other function tests such as Ishihara colour, Amsler chart, pupil reactions, visual fields and eye movements first
- Examine the eye from the front to the back. Start with the periocular area, lids, external eye, cornea, anterior segment, lens, vitreous, macula, retina and optic nerve head, and measure the intraocular pressure

Common eye examination abbreviations

R = right
A/C = anterior chamber
L = left
IOP = intraocular pressure
VA = visual acuity
CT = cover test
UA = unaided
EOM = external ocular movements
PH = pinhole
CDR = cup-disc ratio

Ophthalmology at a Glance, Second Edition. Jane Olver, Lorraine Cassidy, Gurjeet Jutley, and Laura Crawley. © 2014 Jane Olver, Lorraine Cassidy, Gurjeet Jutley and Laura Crawley. Published 2014 by John Wiley & Sons, Ltd. Companion Website: www.ataglanceseries.com/ophthal

You will find that time taken to obtain a good history from the patient is the key to getting the right diagnosis. Whilst you are listening to the patient, you should also observe his or her face and eyes, as much can be gained by simple observation before even measuring the visual acuity and using your ophthalmoscope. Firstly, however, you must introduce yourself and tell the patient what you will be doing.

Aims

- Take a good ophthalmic history.
- Take a thorough medical history.
- Examine the eye in a systematic way.
- Record the eye examination in a standard fashion (Figure 4.1).

Structure of ophthalmic history

Presenting complaint (PC)

You should help the patient by asking *general questions*:

- 'What is the problem with your eyes?'
- 'What do you notice wrong with your vision?' or
- 'Why did your optometrist (or optician) suggest that you be seen in the eye department?'

Sometimes the patient hasn't noticed anything wrong, for instance glaucoma, and is being referred because the optometrist has noticed abnormal discs (possibility of glaucoma) or found an abnormal pigmented lesion in the retina (possibility of melanoma).

Ask *specific questions*:

- Ask if the problem is **acute (e.g. sudden) loss of vision** (see Chapters 18, 19 and 20). Establish which eye is involved or whether the patient thinks it is both eyes. Ask about associated symptoms such as headache, jaw claudication and temporal tenderness. This may help point the direction to a neuro-ophthalmic cause such as temporal arteritis (also called giant cell arteritis; see Chapter 56).
- If the patient says that the problem is **chronic (e.g. slowly developing) bulgy eye (proptosis or exophthalmos)** (see Chapter 29), ask when he or she first noticed it and whether it has changed, such as by getting worse, stabilizing or even getting better.

History of the presenting complaint (HPC)

Some questions to ask include: 'When did the symptom first start?' 'Constant or intermittent?' 'How many attacks or episodes?' 'Any associated features?' 'Getting worse, staying the same or improving?'

Family history (FH)

Ask about eye conditions such as squint, glasses and glaucoma, childhood cataract, ocular tumours or any 'eye disease'.

Past ocular history (POH)

Ask about previous eye problems, eye surgery or 'lazy eye' (amblyopia).

Allergies

Enquire about drug allergies.

Past medical history (PMH)

This is very important in ophthalmology as so many conditions have medical causes. Ask about diabetes, hypertension, irregular heart rate, asthma and chronic obstructive airway disease (COAD), as beta-blockers used in drop form for glaucoma should be avoided in these patients. Other medical conditions, including multiple sclerosis, sarcoid, collagen disorders and inflammatory bowel disease, may present with ophthalmic problems. Enquire about nasal disease such as sinusitis and hay fever, trauma or surgery.

Medications

Some medications may be contraindicated in eye surgery, such as warfarin and aspirin. Some questions to ask include: 'Are you taking any tablets, even homeopathic ones or vitamins?' 'Are you taking aspirin or warfarin?' 'Has your doctor given you any eye drops or creams?' 'Are you taking any other tablets such as hormone replacement therapy?' 'Do you take any tablets for blood pressure or diabetes?'

Social history

Smoking can be a causative factor in retinal and optic nerve vascular occlusive disease. It is a recognized risk factor for thyroid eye disease (Graves ophthalmopathy, discussed in Chapter 30) and for Leber's optic neuropathy (Chapter 53). Some questions to ask include: 'Do you smoke?' 'How many per day?' 'When did you stop?'

The eye examination

Before examining the patient, wash your hands. You can wear disposable gloves if you wish if you think they have an infective conjunctivitis.

A systematic approach is essential. Record your findings pictorially and in a standard way. Always tell the story and have a section for history, then examination, then findings or impression and a written plan. Always write your name, grade and signature at the end.

First measure the visual function.

- Visual acuity. Measure the distance and near vision for each eye separately with their distance and near glasses or contact lens if they wear them. Use the pinhole if the vision is not as good as 6/6 or 20/20 Snellen or 0 on the Logmar chart, which will correct. The pinhole will correct for mild and moderate refractive disorders. Record if the vision was 'unaided' (without glasses or contact lenses) or 'with' (with glasses or contact lenses). Enquire if they have had corneal refractive surgery. If they have had refractive surgery, they may have one eye 'set' for distance and the other for near vision, which is mono-vision or blended mono-vision.
- Visual fields see Chapter 6.
- Colour vision see Chapter 7.

Systematic examination

- Order of examination using slit lamp examination or ophthalmoscope—from front to back of eye.
- Only dilate the pupils once you have done a thorough examination undilated right eye, then left; eyelids; external eye—conjunctiva and fornices; cornea; anterior chamber; lens; vitreous body; retina (optic disc, macula and porterior pole; peripheral retina).

Measure the intraocular pressure and examine the papillary responses.

Only then can you dilate the pupils! Make sure the patient is not driving, as the dilating drops will blur their vision for distance and affect their accommodation. Dilating drops usually take 15–20 minutes to work and the effect may last several hours.

For examination of posterior pole (fundus) see Chapter 11.

> **KEY POINTS**
>
> - Establish if the eye problem is acute or chronic.
> - Medical history is very important.
> - Always measure the visual acuity before dilating the pupils.

Figure 5.1 Snellen charts

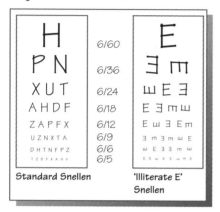

H	6/60
P N	6/36
X U T	6/24
A H D F	6/18
Z A P F X	6/12
U Z N X T A	6/9
D H T N F P Z	6/6
T Z D F X A H V	6/5

Standard Snellen   **'Illiterate E' Snellen**

Figure 5.3 Distance visual acuity test

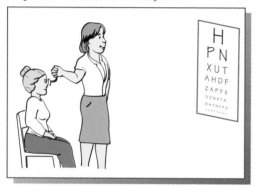

Figure 5.4 Pinhole test

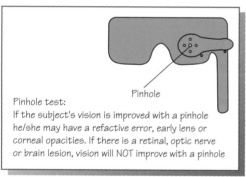

Pinhole

Pinhole test:
If the subject's vision is improved with a pinhole he/she may have a refractive error, early lens or corneal opacities. If there is a retinal, optic nerve or brain lesion, vision will NOT improve with a pinhole

Figure 5.2 (a) and (b) LogMar charts

(a)

VA conversion chart		
UK	USA	Europe (LogMar)
6/6	20/20	0
6/12	20/40	↓
6/36	20/120	
6/60	20/200	1.0
CF	20/400	

Principles of LogMar acuity

The LogMar chart has 10 lines, each with the same number of letters (5 per line). Each letter has an equal value of 0.02 LogMar units. If the patient can read 3 of 5 letters on the line, take the score for the line and add 0.02 per letter not seen (a higher score is worse)

(b)

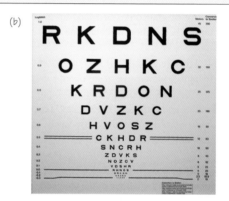

LogMar chart

TIP

If the patient has an artificial eye (AE)/ocular prosthesis record the vision as AE

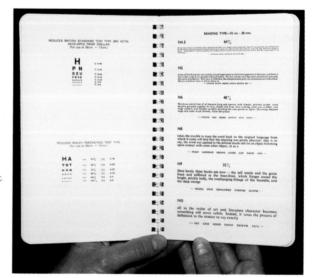

Figure 5.5 Near acuity test

Ophthalmology at a Glance, Second Edition. Jane Olver, Lorraine Cassidy, Gurjeet Jutley, and Laura Crawley. © 2014 Jane Olver, Lorraine Cassidy, Gurjeet Jutley and Laura Crawley. Published 2014 by John Wiley & Sons, Ltd. Companion Website: www.ataglanceseries.com/ophthal

Measurement of visual acuity (VA) is the fundamental measure in ophthalmology and should be done prior to instilling any eye drops. It is important both clinically and medico-legally.

Aims
- Measure distance and near VA.
- Know why and how to use the pinhole test (PH).

Definitions
- **Visual acuity**: an objective measure of what the person can see.
- **Pinhole test**: a simple optical test used to detect the presence of small to moderate refractive errors. (See Chapter 8 for pinhole optics.)

Distance and near vision
VA must be measured, one eye at a time, for both distance and near type, with the patient wearing his or her best spectacle or contact lens correction.
- Test the distance VA first.
- Always start with the right eye.
- If the eyelid is droopy (ptosis), use a finger to lift it gently above the visual axis.
- Insert topical anaesthesia if needed (e.g. if with a painful corneal abrasion and blepharospasm).

The methods of vision testing described here can be used in children 6 years and older, but if an adult or an older child has a severe learning disability, then a method of vision testing appropriate to that individual should be used (see Chapter 22).

> **TIP**
>
> It is important to test both distance and near VA; conditions such as age-related macular degeneration are often disproportionately worse for distance.

Distance vision
- **Snellen acuity (Figure 5.1)**: this is the traditional chart. Snellen vision is measured at 6 m (Europe) or 20 feet (United States).
- **LogMar acuity (Figure 5.2)**: this is increasingly being used for children and patients with poor vision or contrast problems and is useful for research and statistical analysis. The test is done with the patient 4 m from the chart. A LogMar score of 0 is normal, equivalent to 6/6 or 20/20; a score of 1.0 is equivalent to 6/60.

Principles of Snellen acuity
The Snellen chart has letters, but there are also versions with the 'illiterate E' and numbers.
- The 6/6 (20/20) line is 'normal' vision—patients can often read the lower lines, 6/5 or 6/4, which is better than normal.
- The number above the line describes the distance the patient is from the Snellen chart; 6/6 (20/20) means the patient is at 6 m (20 feet).
- The number below the line denotes which line is seen, for example 6/12 (20/40). At 6 m, the patient reads the fifth line down (the '12' line).
- On the 6/6 (20/20) line, each letter is constructed to subtend an angle of 1 minute of arc at a testing distance of 6 m.
- On the 6/18 or 20/60 line, each letter subtends an angle of 3 minutes of arc; the 6/60 (20/200) line, 10 minutes of arc.

- Each line is constructed in a similar way, so that letters on the 6/18 line subtend an angle of 1 minute of arc if tested at 18 m from the chart, and those on the 6/60 line at 60 m from the chart.

How to test distance Snellen VA (Figure 5.3)
- Patient sits 6 m from the chart.
- Distance glasses or contact lenses are worn.
- Occlude one eye *completely* using the palm of the patient's hand or an eye occluder.
- Ask the patient to read down the chart as far as possible.
- Repeat for the other eye.
- Use the pinhole (Figure 5.4, and see Chapter 8) if the VA is less than 6/9. If a refractive error is revealed, this patient needs to be assessed for glasses.
- If the VA is worse than 6/60, even when using the pinhole, move the patient 3 m closer to the chart—if the top line is now read, record the VA as 3/60.
- If the patient cannot see 3/60, sit him or her 1 m from the chart. If the chart still cannot be seen, proceed to measure 'counting fingers' vision. Ask how many fingers are held up, and if the response is accurate, record as **CF (counts fingers)** and the distance measured.
- If CF cannot be seen, move your hand in front of the patient's eye; if movement is accurately seen, record a VA of **HM (hand movements)**, specifying the distance at which movement was seen.
- If hand movements are not perceived, shine a torch light into the eye from various angles and record whether or not the patient has **PL (perception of light)**, from which direction it is perceived, and the distance at which the torch was held.
- If the patient still has no PL, record the vision in that eye as **NPL (no perception of light)**.

> **TIP**
>
> Note: if a patient cannot read, use the illiterate E test (see Figure 5.1). The patient is asked to indicate with hand gestures which way the Es point.

Near vision
How to test near vision
- Ask the patient to wear reading glasses if owned.
- Test each eye separately.
- Patient holds the near test chart (Figure 5.5) at about 0.3 m to read the smallest print that he or she can comfortably see.
- The smallest print is recorded as N4 or N5, and the print increases in increments to the largest, which is N48.
- Some near-reading test types use Jaeger type, which is similar but is recorded as J and the number of the line read.

> **TIP**
>
> N8 is the most common size print in most books.

> **KEY POINTS**
>
> - Test each eye separately.
> - Assess VA before dilating the pupil and before shining a bright light into the eye.
> - Test with a pinhole to detect a refractive error.

6 Examination of visual fields

Figure 6.1 Normal left and right visual fields

The visual fields (left and right, below) are always mapped denoting the left field on the L side of the page and the right field on the R side – in other words the fields are represented as the patient's field actually is as they look at the page. (Have your own fields plotted by the orthoptist in the eye department if she has time, and this way you won't forget!)

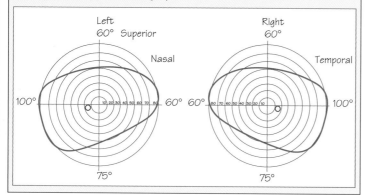

Figure 6.2 Vertical and horizontal ranges of uniocular visual field in degrees. Note that the visual field of each eye overlaps centrally

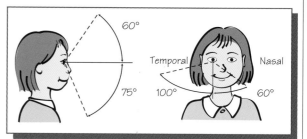

Figure 6.3 How to examine the visual field of each eye separately by confrontation testing. Test each eye separately, starting with the right eye

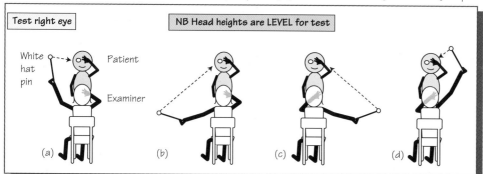

TIP

Some elderly patients, and patients on antiepileptic drugs may have a slightly delayed reaction with confrontation field testing – don't be fooled into thinking they have constricted fields, move the target slowly to allow for this

Figure 6.4 Automated field analyser

In glaucoma screening and management, as in neuro-ophthalmology, the automated visual field analyser provides a reproducible and reliable visual field record. Each eye is tested separately, with the full near lens correction in place if the subject wears reading glasses. A series of lights of variable size and intensity is briefly presented in different locations within the 'bowl' of the perimetry machine, and subjects press the buzzer when they think they see a light, whilst keeping fixation on a central target. Automated perimetry is more sensitive than confrontation visual field testing

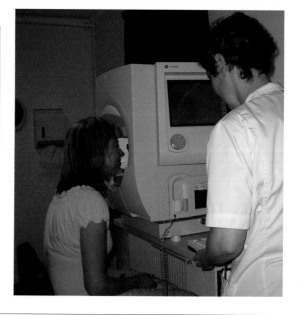

Ophthalmology at a Glance, Second Edition. Jane Olver, Lorraine Cassidy, Gurjeet Jutley, and Laura Crawley. © 2014 Jane Olver, Lorraine Cassidy, Gurjeet Jutley and Laura Crawley. Published 2014 by John Wiley & Sons, Ltd. Companion Website: www.ataglanceseries.com/ophthal

Measurement of the visual fields is also a fundamental test in ophthalmology and should be done prior to instilling any eye drops and with the patient's full refractive error corrected. It is important clinically in patients with glaucoma and in neuro-ophthalmology.

Aim
Examine a visual field by confrontation.

Visual field
The visual field is a map representing the patient's retina, optic nerve and central visual system.
- Test visual fields by **confrontation** for detecting gross abnormalities and neurological problems.
- **Automated static perimetry** is very sensitive and therefore better for detecting more subtle defects such as those seen in early glaucoma (see Chapters 39 and 40).

In your final exam, you may be asked to examine the patient's visual fields by confrontation. You should also be aware of other methods of plotting visual fields, in particular the Goldmann, Humphrey and Esterman automated field analysers. The Esterman binocular visual field is useful for driving licence purposes (see Chapter 3).

Normal field of vision
In individuals with normal, healthy visual pathways, a typical map of the visual field (Figure 6.1) is represented pictorially (Figure 6.2). There is a blind spot temporally in each field—this represents the optic nerve.

> **WARNING**
>
> ▶ A person with poor visual acuity (e.g. as a result of cataract) will have a normal visual field if the visual pathways are intact, but will require a large target in order for his or her fields to be plotted. Don't be fooled into believing that a patient with poor acuity has field loss because you have used a target which is too small—assess visual acuity for near and distance with glasses first.

Examination technique (Figure 6.3)
Necessary equipment for **confrontational field examination**: a white hat pin is best, but a biro with a red cap will do. Red desaturation is an early sign of visual pathway compression.
- Introduce yourself to the patient, and ask him if he would mind you performing an examination of his 'side' or peripheral vision.
- Show the patient the target you will be using, and ask if he can see it at a distance of 0.5 m.
- If the patient cannot see the target at that distance, ask if he can see where your fingers are, and if so use them as your target (as described in the 'TIP' section of this chapter).
- If your fingers are not visible, use a pen torch.
- Sit 1 m in front of the patient with your eyes and the patient's eyes at the same level.

- Always examine the right eye first to avoid any confusion.
- Ask the patient to cover his left eye (make sure it is completely occluded), and if this is not possible, cover the eye with an occluder.
- Ask the patient to look at your left eye and not to look for the target. Explain that you are examining 'side' or peripheral vision, and instruct the patient to say 'yes' whenever he becomes aware of the target in his peripheral vision (or 'out of the corner of his eye'), making sure that his eye gaze is maintained on your left eye at all times.
- Before you start testing peripheral vision with a small target, ask the patient if he can see your face clearly, or if any bits appear to be missing. This will pick up any gross field defects (e.g. if there is a left homonymous hemianopia, the right side of your face will be missing or blurred).
- Now present your target equidistant between yourself and the patient, starting outside the field of vision in the superotemporal quadrant of the visual field (Figure 6.3a), and bring it slowly in towards the centre, keeping the target equidistant between yourself and the patient at all times.
- Maintain fixation on the patient's right eye and make a mental note of when you first see the target in your peripheral field; compare this with when the patient can first see the target. You should both become aware of the target at the same time if there is no field defect.
- Now repeat in the (Figure 6.3b) inferotemporal, (Figure 6.3c) inferonasal and (Figure 6.3d) superonasal quadrants.

> **TIP**
>
> An alternative method that can be used if the patient's acuity is too poor to visualize the target is to present one, three or four fingers in each quadrant of the visual field while the patient looks straight ahead (avoid two fingers so as not to offend). Ask the patient how many digits he can see out of the corner of his eye (vary the number of fingers in each quadrant).

- **Check the blind spot** (note: if the patient has an obvious homonymous hemianopia, altitudinal field defect, bitemporal hemianopia or grossly constricted fields, there is no need to assess the blind spot). Examine one eye at a time. Ensure stable eye fixation at all times. *Slowly* bring a small target (a hat pin is best here) from the centre, on a straight line towards the temporal periphery. Ask the patient to indicate when the top of the hat pin disappears and when it reappears. Compare with your own blind spot.
- Now examine the left field.

> **KEY POINTS**
>
> - Confrontation visual field tests are good for marked field defects, but they are unlikely to detect subtle field changes.
> - Goldmann fields are best for neurological defects.
> - Automated perimetry is best to detect and monitor glaucomatous field defects (Figure 6.4).

7 Other visual functions

Figure 7.1 (a) Photographic representation of the left posterior pole; the optic nerve transmits all retinal nerve fibres centrally, and the macula has dense cones. (b) Schematic representation of the right posterior pole; there are 6 million cones at the posterior pole, and the macula has almost 200 000 cones responsible for colour vision. *Copyright S Downes*

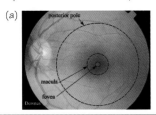

(a)

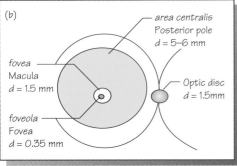

(b)

- area centralis Posterior pole *d* = 5–6 mm
- fovea Macula *d* = 1.5 mm
- foveola Fovea *d* = 0.35 mm
- Optic disc *d* = 1.5mm

Figure 7.2 (a) The book of Ishihara plates, (b) example plates and (c) Ishihara plate testing

Colour vision testing is a NEAR VISION TEST - patient must have their reading spectacles on
Do colour vision tests before shining a bright light in the patient's eyes and before dilating their pupils

(a)

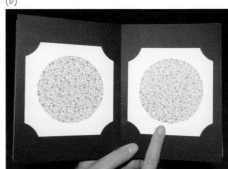

(b)

(c)

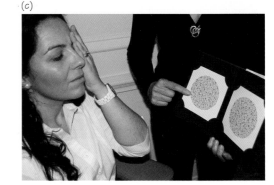

Figure 7.3 (a) The area of the eye tested by the Amsler chart (the central 20Y), (b) an example of an Amsler chart and (c) the appearance of the Amsler chart in a patient with dry age-related macular degeneration – the central lines are distorted due to the maculopathy

(a)

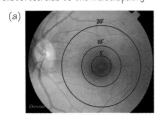

(b) Amsler chart

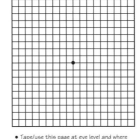

The Amsler chart is a grid given to patients with dry age-related macular degeneration (AMD) to take home and look at regularly. If the lines on the grid become wavy or distorted in a new place this may indicate that the patient has developed a leaky or bleeding subretinal neovascular membrane. This needs urgent assessment to decide suitability for laser treatment

- Tape/use this page at eye level and where light is consistent and without glare
- ALWAYS KEEP THE AMSLER CHART THE SAME DISTANCE FROM YOUR EYES EACH TIME YOU TEST
- Put on your reading glasses and cover one eye
- Fix your gaze on the centre black dot
- Keeping your gaze fixed, try to see if any lines are distorted or missing
- Mark the defect on the chart with a pen
- TEST EACH EYE SEPARATELY
- If the distortion is new to you or has worsened, arrange to see your ophthalmologist at once

(c)

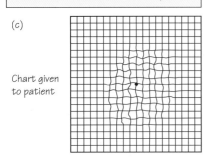

Chart given to patient

TIP

If the patient has reading glasses they should wear them for the colour and Amsler testing

Figure 7.4 The swinging flashlight test

Pupil testing in left optic neuropathy by swinging flashlight test

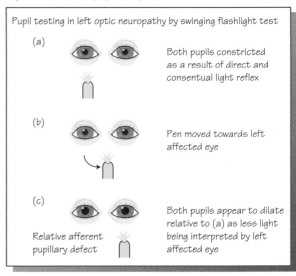

(a) Both pupils constricted as a result of direct and consensual light reflex

(b) Pen moved towards left affected eye

(c) Both pupils appear to dilate relative to (a) as less light being interpreted by left affected eye

Relative afferent pupillary defect

Ophthalmology at a Glance, Second Edition. Jane Olver, Lorraine Cassidy, Gurjeet Jutley, and Laura Crawley. © 2014 Jane Olver, Lorraine Cassidy, Gurjeet Jutley and Laura Crawley. Published 2014 by John Wiley & Sons, Ltd. Companion Website: www.ataglanceseries.com/ophthal

In order to test the visual function, you have to perform three commonly used tests: the Ishihara colour plates, the Amsler grid and pupil reactions. Visual function is dependent on a healthy retina with healthy cones at the macula for colour vision and fine clear detail, and on the optic nerve fibres to convey the visual information to the visual centres.

Aims
• Assess optic nerve function by testing (i) colour vision and (ii) pupil reactions.
• Assess macular function using the Amsler chart.

Colour vision
Colour vision is detected by cones at the macula (Figure 7.1) and is transmitted centrally via the optic nerve. It is a sensitive indicator of optic nerve function, and it is vital to assess when there is anterior visual pathway disease. It is also an indicator of central retinal (cone) function.

Optic nerve
• Colour vision is a test of anterior visual pathway function—mainly of the optic nerve.
• In optic neuritis (which may be associated with multiple sclerosis), papilloedema, optic nerve compression from tumour or Graves' ophthalmopathy or any optic neuropathy, visual acuity may be normal and *only colour vision is affected*.
• Acquired colour vision defects will be noticed by the patient, and they may be asymmetric. Note that a lesion compressing the optic chiasm may cause bilateral colour vision defects, is usually associated with a visual field defect and may progress.

Macula
• Macular disease due to involvement of the cones, either congenital or acquired, causes a disturbance of colour vision.
• An X-linked anomaly of the retinal cones in males will lead to red–green 'colour anomaly' or confusion. This is the common form of 'colour blindness'.

Clinical assessment
Ishihara
• Assess colour vision using pseudo-isochromatic 'Ishihara plates'—a booklet of plates held at the normal reading distance (Figure 7.2a). Each plate has a series of various sized colour dots arranged in patterns of hues to represent numbers (Figure 7.2b). Red and green cone function is predominantly tested by this test.
• The numbers are large to aid people with poor vision.
• The first plate is a 'test plate', which identifies subjects whose reading skills or acuity levels exclude them from taking the test.
• Ask the patient to read each plate, testing each eye separately to exclude a uni-ocular problem (Figure 7.2c).
• There are up to 17 plates of numbers; record colour vision as '17/17' if the patient reads all 17 plates, or '5/17' if she could read only five, or 'test plate only' if she could read only the test plate.
• If the patient cannot read, ask her to trace the coloured pattern on the illiterate plates with her finger.

Red desaturation
Colour vision can be estimated by the patient looking at a red object (e.g. a red pen) with each eye. If there is an optic nerve or tract lesion on one side, the colour looks pink, dull or washed out with that eye. This is 'red desaturation'.

Amsler chart (Figure 7.3)
This chart (Figure 7.3b) is a test of macular function and is useful for picking up subtle paracentral scotomas seen in macular disease (e.g. age-related macular degeneration).
• Ask the patient to hold the grid at arm's length and to fixate on the central black dot.
• Test each eye separately.
• The patient must note whether or not the black lines look distorted (metamorphopsia) or absent (scotoma) (Figure 7.3c).
• Ask the patient to draw in the area of the distortion or missing area.

Pupil reactions
The pupil reactions to a **direct torch light (light response)** and to **accommodation (near response)** are important to exclude optic nerve and neurological disease. (See also Chapter 52 for pupil abnormalities.)

WARNING
▶ If there is gross retinal disease, the direct pupil reactions will also be abnormal due to retinal nerve fibre damage.

• **Direct light response**: tests gross retinal and optic nerve function.
  ○ Sit opposite patient at arm's length.
  ○ Ask the patient to look past you into the distance (avoids accommodative reaction).
  ○ Shine a pen torch light into one eye and assess pupil constriction—the **direct pupil light response**. The **consensual reflex** is the simultaneous constriction of the other pupil.
  ○ Repeat in the other eye.
• **Swinging flashlight test (Figure 7.4)**: this is to detect a relative afferent pupil defect (RAPD), which would be a sign of optic nerve damage.
  ○ Swing the light quickly back to the first eye, with the patient still looking into the distance—the first pupil should constrict, and the second equally constrict.
  ○ Repeat swinging the torch quickly from eye to eye to double check.
  ○ If one pupil dilates instead of constricts, this is an afferent pupil defect indicating a serious retinal or optic nerve problem.
  ○ Always ensure you use the brightest light source available when looking for a RAPD because abnormalities can be subtle.
• **Accommodation (near response)**: this is to test for neurological diseases.
  ○ Ask the patient to look from the distance fixation to a small accommodative target brought towards her slowly, up to a distance of about 20 cm.
  ○ Both pupils should constrict equally.

KEY POINTS
• Ishihara plates measure colour vision.
• The Amsler grid tests central macular function.
• The swinging flashlight test detects afferent pupil defect.

8 Basic optics and refraction

Figure 8.1 Retinoscopy

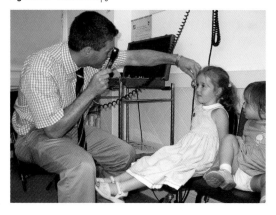

Figure 8.2 Accommodation

A retinoscope is used to measure the refractive error of the eye, in conjunction with lenses from a trial lens set. In children the eyes are first dilated with cyclopentolate drops to inhibit the lens accommodation, but in adults this is not necessary. The spherical and cylindrical ametropia can be measured accurately with retinoscopy. Automated refractometers also exist

Accommodation

- The ciliary body relaxes and the lens becomes fatter

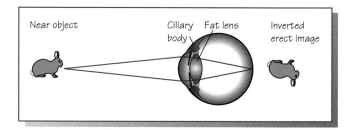

Figure 8.3 Emmetropia, myopia and hypermetropia

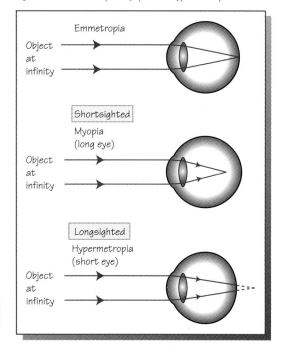

Figure 8.4 The pinhole test

- In emmetropia (more detail in Chapter 9) every point in an object of regard is brought to point focus on the retina and the sum of all the points yields a clear image, i.e. *point-to-point correspondence*

- If there is a refractive error present, a blur circle is formed on the retina, which is dependent on the size of their pupil (smaller pupil = smaller blur circle)

- When a pinhole aperture is placed in front of the eye, it acts as an artificial small pupil and the size of the blur circle is abolished/reduced, producing a clearer image

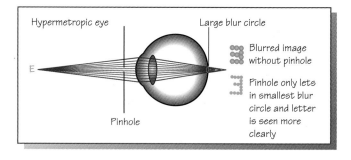

Refractive errors are the commonest ocular problem worldwide. In order to understand the aims of cataract surgery, refractive surgery and strabismus surgery, you should understand the basic refractive errors. With the increasing ageing population, presbyopia and its correction by glasses or refractive surgery are becoming bigger issues that need addressing.

Aims

- Refractive errors:
  - What is longsightedness?
  - What is shortsightedness?
  - What is astigmatism?
- Accommodative changes with age.

This chapter summarizes the basic optics of the eye and defines refraction.

Refraction by the eye

- The ability of the eye to bend light rays.
- Determined by the refractive media (cornea and lens) plus the axial length of the eye.
- Refraction is calculated in dioptres (D) (e.g. 1D is the power of a convergent lens to focus parallel light at its focal point (f) 1 m behind the lens).
- The total refractive power of an emmetropic eye (normal length) is approximately 58D, of which 43D is contributed by the cornea and 15D by the lens, the aqueous and the vitreous.

Refraction techniques

These are techniques for testing the refraction of the eye.

Subjective refraction

The patient distinguishes between the effects of various lenses on the visibility of letters on the Snellen and LogMar charts.

Objective refraction

This includes examination with the ophthalmoscope, the retinoscope or various types of autorefractors.

Retinoscopy

- This technique is particularly useful in testing children under 7 years for glasses.
- In children under 7 years old, retinoscopy must be done with cycloplegia (drops inserted to temporarily paralyse the ciliary body and inhibit accommodation; see Chapter 12) in order to obtain an accurate refraction.
- A retinoscope is an instrument used to assess the **objective** refraction of the eye. A bright streak of light is shone through the pupil and is seen as a red reflex reflected from the retina (Figure 8.1).
- The retinoscope streak is moved gently, and the direction of the light reflex from the retina is observed.
- By placing a series of plus or minus lenses in front of the patient's eye, the observer can calculate whether the patient is shortsighted (myopic) or longsighted (hypermetropic) and measure the amount of astigmatism that needs correcting.

Accommodation (Figure 8.2)

The ability of the eye to focus clearly on an object at any distance is due to the elasticity of the lens. The **far point** is the furthest distance away at which an object can be seen clearly. In order to see a near object clearly, the ciliary muscle must relax (a parasympathetic reaction), enabling the lens to become fatter and bend (refract) the light rays more, so that they are in focus on the retina. The nearest point that the eye can see clearly with maximum accommodation in force is called the **near point**. The distance between these two points is the **range of accommodation**. See presbyopia in the 'Refractive Errors' section of this chapter!

Emmetropia = normal eye with no refractive error

Light from sources beyond 5 m is focused by the non-accommodating eye as a sharp but inverted image on the fovea. The brain interprets this as a clear, upright image.

Refractive errors (Figure 8.3)

For correction of refractive errors, see Chapter 9.

- **Hypermetropia**: longsightedness. Patient can see clearly in the distance but not near.

  Optics: the focal point is behind the retina. The converging rays that fall on the retina produce a blurred image.

  Cause: the axial length is too short.

  Correction: convex (plus) glasses

- **Myopia**: shortsightedness. Patients can see clearly close up, but their distance vision is blurred.

  Optics: the focal point is in front of the retina. Divergent light rays falling on the retina produce a blurred image.

  Cause: most commonly, excessive axial length (axial myopia); rarely due to too great refractive power (e.g. cataract refractive myopia).

  Correction: concave (minus) glasses.

- **Astigmatism**: part of the image in one plane is out of focus due to unequal refraction.

  Optics: the parallel incoming rays deform and do not focus at a single point, causing a blurred retinal image.

  Cause: corneal curvature.

  Correction: cylinders (toric lenses), corneal surgery or laser surgery.

- **Presbyopia**: gradual loss of focusing power. The subject is usually over 45 years old and cannot see clearly to read near type. They progressively hold the type further and further away until their arms no longer reach far enough.

  Optics: there is a normal loss of accommodative range with increasing age, due to a decline of lens elasticity.

  Cause: stiffening of lens and weaking of the ciliary body muscle.

  Correction: the reading correction (plus sphere) is added to the distance correction.

Refractive errors are increasingly being corrected by laser refractive surgery, see Chapter 35

KEY POINTS

- The refractive power of the eye is largely due to the cornea and lens.
- Myopic eyes have a long axial length; hypermetropic eyes have a short axial length.
- Presbyopia is when reading text blurs due to changes in accommodation at around age 45 years.

9 Glasses, contact lenses and low-vision aids

Figure 9.1 Correction of refractive errors

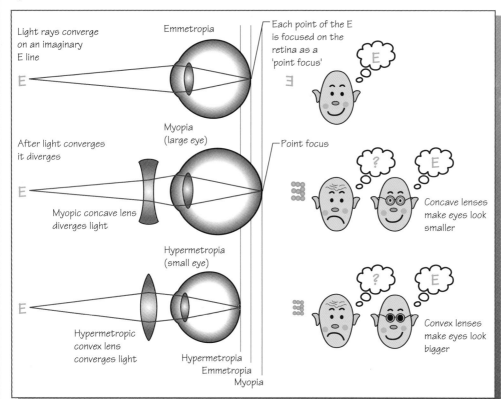

Light rays converge on an imaginary E line

After light converges it diverges

Emmetropia

Myopia (large eye)

Myopic concave lens diverges light

Hypermetropia (small eye)

Hypermetropic convex lens converges light

Hypermetropia
Emmetropia
Myopia

Each point of the E is focused on the retina as a 'point focus'

Point focus

Concave lenses make eyes look smaller

Convex lenses make eyes look bigger

Figure 9.2 (a) Contact lenses, (b) biconcave shape for myopia, (c) biconvex shape for presbyopia and hypermetropia and (d) prism shape for diplopia

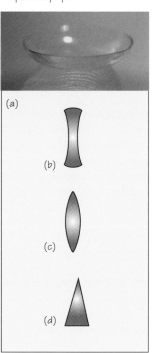

(a)

(b)

(c)

(d)

Figure 9.3 Low-vision aids. (a) Handheld magnification devices, (b) spectacles with magnifying aids, (c) close-circuit television (CCTV) and (d) scrolling with CCTV. *Copyright S Downes*

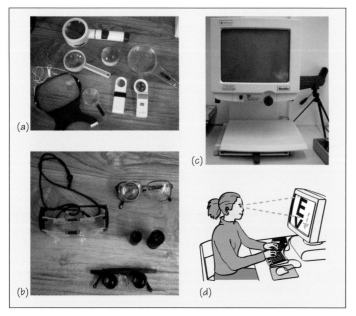

(a)

(b)

(c)

(d)

Figure 9.4 (a) Fresnel prism and (b) Fresnel stuck on right lens

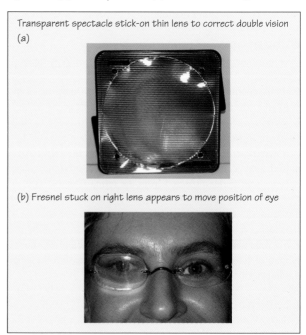

Transparent spectacle stick-on thin lens to correct double vision
(a)

(b) Fresnel stuck on right lens appears to move position of eye

Although many people are having corneal refractive surgery to correct their refractive error, glasses and contact lenses remain the first choice for the majority. Low-vision aids can help both young adults in employment with inherited macular disorders, and older people with age-related macular degeneration.

Aims
- Correction of refractive errors with glasses and contact lenses.
- Types of contact lenses.
- Use of low-vision aids.

For laser refractive surgery, see Chapter 35.

Optical lenses (Figure 9.1)
Spherical lens
This lens has an equal curvature in all meridians.
- Concave (minus) lens:
  - Used to correct myopia.
  - Refracts light rays, making them more divergent.
  - Objects seen through a minus lens look smaller.
- Convex (plus) lens:
  - Used to correct hypermetropia, presbyopia and aphakia.
  - Refracts light rays to make them more convergent.
  - Objects seen through a plus lens look larger.

Toric (cylinder) lens
- Used to correct astigmatism.
- Shaped like a section through a rugby ball with one meridian more curved than the other (at right angles to each other).

Prisms
- A prism deviates light rays.
- Used to relieve diplopia by redirecting light onto the fovea.
- Fresnel prisms are temporary plastic prisms that are stuck onto the patient's glasses to join diplopia (e.g. sixth cranial nerve palsy).

Contact lenses (CLs) (Figure 9.2)
- CLs are superior in severe refractive errors and give better quality vision (e.g. correction of aphakia where an intraocular lens has not been placed is best corrected with a convex CL).
- Also used *therapeutically* in corneal disease as bandage CLs or as cosmetic lenses for the scarred cornea. See Chapter 34.

Indications for CLs
- Cosmetic (e.g. avoid glasses in low myopia).
- For sport (e.g. tennis and skiing for wider field).
- Severe refractive errors:
  - High myopia (e.g. >6D myopia): a patient with high myopia depends on contact lenses for visual acuity and a wider visual field.
  - Aphakic children without an intraocular lens post-congenital cataract surgery.
  - Irregular astigmatism (e.g. rigid contact lenses for **corneal scarring** and **keratoconus**). In the later stages, surgery (penetrating keratoplasty) may be required (see Chapter 32).

Types of CLs
Hard or rigid CLs
- Polymethylmethacrylate (PMMA).
- Poor oxygen transmission.

Soft CLs
- Hydroxymethylmethacrylate (HMMA).
- Better oxygen permeability but fragile.
- The most common type of contact lenses worn for simple refractive errors and as bandage contact lenses.

Disposable soft CLs
- Disposable lens are replaced daily, weekly or monthly.
- Disadvantage: higher infection rate (e.g. acanthamoeba).

Extended-wear soft CLs
- Risk of overwear syndrome.
- Complications more common (see Chapter 34).

Coloured or tinted CLs (soft or hard-rigid)
These are used for prosthetic purposes as hand-painted iris-coloured lenses:
- Cover corneal opacities, iris defects or cataracts in blind eyes.
- Prevent photophobia and improve vision in aniridia and albinism.

Rigid gas-permeable CLs
- Made from a mixture of hard and soft CL materials.
- Transmit oxygen much better than PMMA.
- Good for patients who are allergic to soft CLs.

Scleral lenses
- A type of hard CL approximately 23 mm in diameter that bridges the corneoscleral junction.
- Used for prosthesis purposes and keratoconus.

Low-vision aids
Important in the **visual rehabilitation** of patients with central visual field loss, especially macular degeneration.

Text magnification
Optical magnification with **magnifiers** (Figure 9.3a) and **telescopic glasses** (Figure 9.3b):
- Magnifiers increase the image at least 4× the normal size.
- Telescopic glasses increase the image size at least 8×, but cause constriction of the visual field.
- Closed-circuit television (CCTV) systems (Figure 9.3c) allow a magnification of 25× and are beneficial for patients with a high degree of vision loss. However, these are expensive!

Page navigation
In patients with macular degeneration, fixation stability is often very poor and they have chaotic reading eye movements using a lot of searching with small saccades. This can be improved by encouraging non-foveal reading.
- Eccentric vision training.
- New methods of presenting text, such as electronic scrolled text (i.e. move text to them or serial presentation on a TV screen).
- High-tech magnification and image enhancement using a head-mounted CCTV with image processing of contrast enhancement (virtual reality).

> **KEY POINTS**
> - Glasses' correction of myopia reduces the size of the image.
> - Contact lenses' correction of myopia gives a larger visual field than glasses.
> - Fresnel prisms (Figure 9.4) are stuck onto glasses to correct diplopia.

Figure 10.1 Diagrams of (a) the external eye, (b) the anterior segment and (c) the eyelids

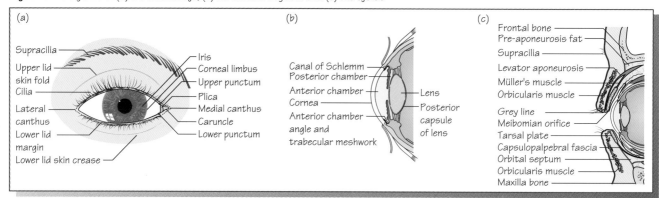

(a)

Supracilia
Upper lid skin fold
Cilia
Lateral canthus
Lower lid margin
Lower lid skin crease
Iris
Corneal limbus
Upper punctum
Plica
Medial canthus
Caruncle
Lower punctum

(b)

Canal of Schlemm
Posterior chamber
Anterior chamber
Cornea
Anterior chamber angle and trabecular meshwork
Lens
Posterior capsule of lens

(c)

Frontal bone
Pre-aponeurosis fat
Supracilia
Levator aponeurosis
Müller's muscle
Orbicularis muscle
Grey line
Meibomian orifice
Tarsal plate
Capsulopalpebral fascia
Orbital septum
Orbicularis muscle
Maxilla bone

Figure 10.2 How to evert an upper eyelid

Place a cotton bud or Minims gently on the upper lid skin crease, hold the central eyelashes and draw them upwards, at the same time pressing gently downwards with the cotton bud/Minims as counter pressure. Ask the patient to look downwards as this makes it more comfortable. Topical anaesthetic drops are recommended to anaesthetize the ocular surface as everting the eyelid can be uncomfortable. See Chapter 12, use of eye drops

Direct visual assessment with adequate magnification and illumination is required, using a loup and pen torch, direct ophthalmoscope or slit lamp

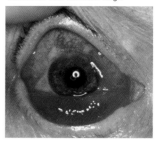

Figure 10.3 Gross conjunctival chemosis and haemorrhage

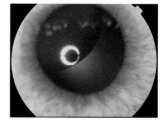

Figure 10.4 Dislocated lens

Figure 10.5 Corneal abrasion staining with fluorescein (see Chapter 17)

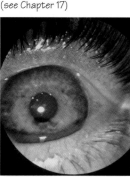

Figure 10.6 Goldmann tonometry to measure intraocular pressure (see Chapter 40)

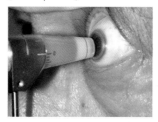

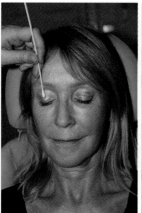

Figure 10.7 Using the slit lamp (see Chapter 11)

Slit lamp

This provides the best magnification and illumination with a stereoscopic view. The Goldmann tonometer can be attached to it to measure intraocular pressure and a variety of hand-held lenses used with it to view the fundus

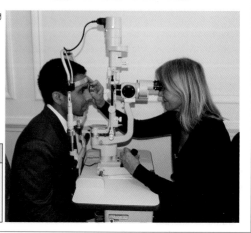

Ophthalmology at a Glance, Second Edition. Jane Olver, Lorraine Cassidy, Gurjeet Jutley, and Laura Crawley. © 2014 Jane Olver, Lorraine Cassidy, Gurjeet Jutley and Laura Crawley. Published 2014 by John Wiley & Sons, Ltd. Companion Website: www.ataglanceseries.com/ophthal

Ophthalmic examination requires a basic knowledge of the anatomy of the eyelids and front of the eye. You should perform direct observation unaided, with a loup and torch, or with an ophthalmoscope, followed by slit lamp examination.

Aims
• Anatomy of the external eye and anterior segment.
• Examination.

Anatomy
The **external eye** (Figure 10.1a) includes the eyelids (Figure 10.1c), lashes, lacrimal puncta, caruncle, plica semilunaris, corneal epithelium and conjunctiva.

The **anterior segment** (Figure 10.1b) includes the cornea, iris, anterior chamber angle and lens.

Systematic examination
This should be undertaken in the following order.

Lids
• Observe the **upper eyelids** for **symmetry**. If asymmetrical, decide which lid is ptotic (drooping) or whether the other lid is retracted.
• Observe the lid position relative to the pupil and cornea.
• A ptotic lid will cover more cornea and may partially or totally obscure the pupil.
• A retracted lid will cover little or no cornea, with the sclera visible above the cornea (upper scleral show).
• Observe the **lower eyelid position** for entropion (lid turning inwards) or ectropion (lid everted outwards).
• Look for evidence of **inflammation** (e.g. erythema or oedema).
• Note any **lid lesions** present.
• Observe the **eyelashes**—any missing? Are they growing in the correct direction or in-growing (trichiasis)?
• When appropriate, **evert the eyelid** (Figure 10.2).

Conjunctiva
• Use the slit lamp at low (10×) magnification, a pen torch or an ophthalmoscope set at +12D held close to the eye or set to zero and held further away.
• **Colour**:
  ◦ Red (Figure 10.3). Is there injection (i.e. redness?). Does it involve the entire conjunctival surface, a segment of conjunctiva or just the area where the conjunctiva meets the cornea (circumciliary)?
  ◦ Bluish or purple circumciliary injection suggests anterior uveitis.
  ◦ In chemical burns, patches of ischaemia appear white, surrounded by severe congestion (see Chapter 16).
  ◦ Yellow. Patients with jaundice may have a yellow tinge to their conjunctiva (icterus).
• **Appearance and texture** of the conjunctiva:
  ◦ Are there tarsal conjunctival follicles or papillae? These are pinkish or fine red velvety lumps.
  ◦ Does the patient have chemosis (conjunctiva has an oedematous jelly-like appearance)?

Cornea
Use the same equipment as when examining the conjunctiva.
• Is the cornea clear, or are opacities present?
• If there is a corneal irregularity or opacity, instil a drop of fluorescein into the conjunctival sac and note any fluorescein uptake (i.e. staining),

which indicates a break in the epithelium (Figure 10.5). A blue torch light is best.
• Are there abnormal vessels (neovascularization) growing into the cornea? It should be avascular.

Intraocular pressure (IOP)
For eye pressure measurement, see Figure 10.6 and Chapter 37.

Anterior chamber (AC)
Information about the AC is best obtained with the slit lamp (Figure 10.7). The direct ophthalmoscope (set at +10D) or a pen torch and loup will provide useful but limited information.
• Is the AC quiet (i.e. is the aqueous clear?)? A slit lamp will show the presence of cells and keratoprecipitates (KPs) (condensation of cells on the inner surface of the cornea).
• Is there a hyphaema (accumulation of blood in the AC)? This may result from trauma, spontaneously ruptured iris new vessels (rubeosis iridis) with a central retinal vein occlusion, longstanding glaucoma or diabetic retinopathy, or in patients with intraocular tumours.

WARNING

▶ Beware the child with a hyphaema and no history of trauma—think of retinoblastoma or non-accidental injury.

• Is there a hypopyon (accumulation of white blood cells in the AC)? This may be seen in uveitis, in infective endophthalmitis, with a corneal abscess and as a manifestation of leukaemia or lymphoma.

Iris
Use the slit lamp, the ophthalmoscope at +8D or the pen torch and loup.
• Notice the colour of each iris. Different colour irides ('iris heterochromia') may be associated with iritis or congenital Horner's syndrome.
• Identify iris lesions: iris melanoma, Lisch nodules in neurofibromatosis or abnormal iris vessels (rubeosis irides), which may signify an underlying ocular tumour, central retinal vein occlusion or diabetes.
• Notice iatrogenic iris changes (e.g. peripheral iridectomy).

Lens
The slit lamp or direct ophthalmoscope is best to examine the lens.
• Use the direct ophthalmoscope set at 0, and stand at arm's length from the patient, directing the beam of light to the pupil to assess the red reflex. Lens opacities are seen as specs in the red reflex.
• Next, move closer to the patient, at the same time increasing the magnification (usually to +6) until the lens is in focus.
• Detect a dislocated lens (Figure 10.4) with the pupil dilated. It may be caused by trauma or may indicate an underlying hereditary systemic disorder such as Marfan's syndrome or homocystinuria.

KEY POINTS

• Examine the eye systematically, starting with the eyelids, the external eye and anterior segment.
• The cornea is usually avascular with a shiny smooth surface.
• Cataract is the most common lens disorder.

---

11 Posterior segment and retina

Figure 11.1 Posterior pole anatomy

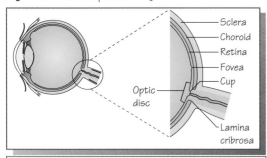

Sclera
Choroid
Retina
Fovea
Cup
Optic disc
Lamina cribrosa

The optic nerve head consists of approximately 1.3 million axons exiting the globe via the lamina cribrosa at the posterior scleral foramen (small hole in the back of the sclera). The neural rim (pink) contains axons and the central cup (yellow), glial tissue

Figure 11.2 The layers of the retina

Tight junction
Choriocapillaris
Bruch's membrane
Horizontal cell
Retinal pigment epithelium
Photoreceptors
Outer segments
External limiting membrane
Outer nuclear layer
Outer plexiform layer
Inner nuclear layer
Inner plexiform layer
Ganglion cell layer
Nerve fibre layer
Internal limiting membrane

Figure 11.3 Direct ophthalmoscope

The hand-held ophthalmoscope is commonly used in clinical medicine to view the pupil reactions, red reflex, lens, retina and optic nerve head, even through an undilated pupil. It has a monocular view

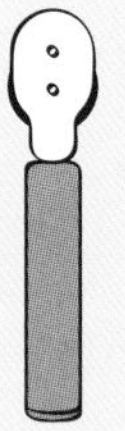

Figure 11.4 Normal optic disc

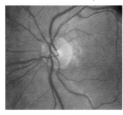

Figure 11.5 Central retinal artery occlusion. There is a pale retina, occluded arterioles and a cherry red spot

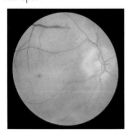

Figure 11.6 Central retinal vein occlusion. There is a swollen disc with marked venous engorgement and haemorrhages

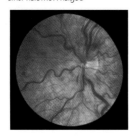

Figure 11.9 Indirect ophthalmoscope

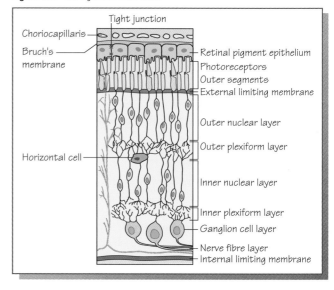

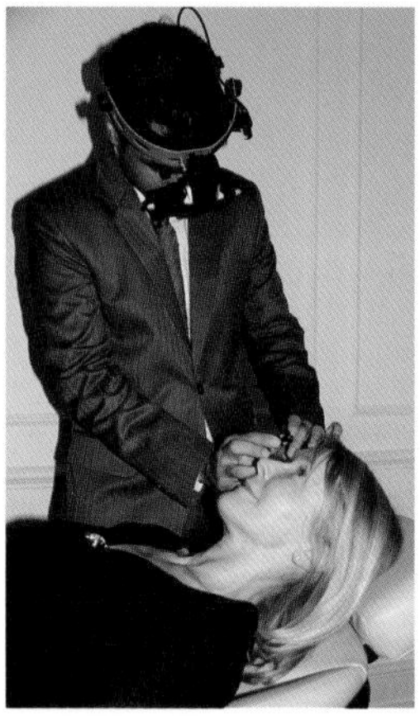

Figure 11.10 Fundus lenses; digital high magnification lens and digital wide-field lens

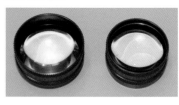

Figure 11.7 Yellow drusen in Bruch's membrane (age-related changes) at macula in age-related macular degeneration (AMD)

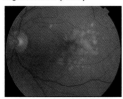

Figure 11.8 Laser at macula: small, regular, pale laser burns in retina

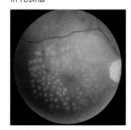

Special lenses are held in front of the patient's eye to view the disc and macula at high magnification – the image seen is inverted and horizontally transposed

Figure 11.11 Slit lamp

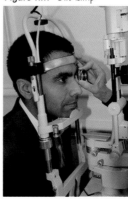

Figure 11.12 The amount of the retina that can be seen with direct and indirect ophthalmoscopy and the slit lamp technique

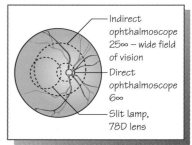

Indirect ophthalmoscope 25∞ – wide field of vision
Direct ophthalmoscope 6∞
Slit lamp, 78D lens

Ophthalmology at a Glance, Second Edition. Jane Olver, Lorraine Cassidy, Gurjeet Jutley, and Laura Crawley. © 2014 Jane Olver, Lorraine Cassidy, Gurjeet Jutley and Laura Crawley. Published 2014 by John Wiley & Sons, Ltd. Companion Website: www.ataglanceseries.com/ophthal

The ophthalmologist is skilful in examining the fundus. You too should learn the posterior segment anatomy and be able to confidently use a direct ophthalmoscope, even without a dilated pupil.

Aims
- Define the fundus.
- Understand how to use an ophthalmoscope to examine the fundus.
- Attempt the use of (i) an indirect ophthalmoscope, and (ii) a slit lamp plus special lenses.

Direct ophthalmoscopy is an essential skill since retinal examination is widely used in general practice and hospital medicine.

Definitions
- **Fundus**: the retina, including the macula, blood vessels and optic nerve head.
- **Posterior segment**: the area behind the lens, including the posterior chamber, vitreous, retina, choroid and optic disc.
- **Fundoscopy**: examination of the fundus.
- **Posterior pole (Figure 11.1)**: the posterior retina, including the optic nerve head, macula and retinal blood vessels.
- **Periphery or peripheral fundus**: the retina (Figure 11.2 and Appendix 2) from the equator out towards the pars plana.

Examination technique
Equipment needed to examine posterior segment:
- **Direct ophthalmoscope**: monocular.
- **Indirect ophthalmoscope**: binocular; with a 20D lens.
- **Slit lamp biomicroscope**: binocular; with or without a +90D or +78D lens.

Dilate the pupils for a better view
- The fundus can be examined with the pupil undilated (best in darkness to ensure maximum pupil size). A better view is achieved if the pupils are dilated.
- In adults, Guttae (g) tropicamide 1% is used. Phenylephrine hydrochloride (G 55) 2.5% or 10% can be given for greater dilation, especially with brown irides (see Chapter 12).

Do not dilate the pupils in the following situations
- When responses are being monitored for neuro-observation (such as to assess a relative afferent pupillary defect).
- When there is a risk of precipitating angle-closure glaucoma (i.e. individuals with shallow anterior angles) (see Chapter 39).

Direct ophthalmoscopy
The light source is focussed by a series of mini-lenses and directed via a mirror into the patient's eye (Figure 11.3). The observer views the illuminated retina through a sight hole in the mirror. The disc of rotating lenses can be rotated to compensate for both the observer's and patient's refractive errors—if both the observer and patient are emmetropic, then no lens (zero) is incorporated. The image produced is virtual and erect (i.e. the right way up). and it is magnified (15×) with a field of view of 6° (Figure 11.12).

How to use the direct ophthalmoscope
If you wear glasses or contact lenses for distance. keep them on. Note: start with the ophthalmoscope magnification set at 0.
- Ask the patient to look straight ahead.
  - Emphasize the importance of looking into the distance to avoid accommodation (and thus constricting the pupils and making your life harder!).
- Use your right eye to examine the patient's right eye first: then repeat the examination of the left eye using your left eye.
  - Stand or sit at arm's length, looking through the ophthalmoscope aperture.
  - Move closer to the patient, looking at the red reflex until the retinal details become clear, with the patient continually looking over your right shoulder into the distance.
- Examine the optic nerve head or disc:
  - Disc margins should be clearly defined and distinct from the surrounding tissue (Figure 11.4).
  - The cup–disc ratio (CDR) is the ratio of the size of the central yellow cup to the size of the entire disc. Whilst variation exists, normalcy should be gauged if observing symmetry to the other side and a CDR less than 0.5.
  - Disc colour: suspect optic atrophy if the disc is completely yellow or white.
- Follow the blood vessels out from the disc in their four directions:
  - Calibre:
    — Are the arteries excessively narrowed as in arteriosclerosis (Figure 11.5)?
    — Are the veins tortuous and dilated as in venous occlusion (Figure 11.6) or ocular ischaemia?
  - Arteriovenous (AV) nipping, which occurs in hypertension and arteriosclerosis.
  - Any other abnormalities (e.g. arteriovenous malformation (AVM), new vessel formation or sheathing).
- Ask the patient to look up, down, right and left, to examine as much of the equatorial retina as possible.
  - Colour—retinal colour can vary between races.
  - Contour—are there any elevated lesions such as metastases, malignant melanoma or retinoblastoma?
- Lastly, ask the patient to look straight at the ophthalmoscope light beam to examine the vessel-free macula and fovea.
  - Fovea is avascular, and there is a sheen from a healthy young fovea.
  - Look for haemorrhages (Figure 11.6), drusen (Figure 11.7), laser scars (Figure 11.8), exudates, oedema or the like.

Indirect ophthalmoscopy (Figure 11.9)
This binocular head-mounted device with hand-held condensing lenses is used to examine the retina binocularly. It gives a wide field of view at low magnification. The image is both upside down and back to front.

Slit lamp biomicroscope (Figures 11.10 and 11.11)
This is predominantly used by ophthalmologists for ophthalmic examination. The retinal image is both upside down and back to front.

KEY POINTS
- Examine the right eye first.
- The optic nerve cup–disc ratio is normally less than 0.5.
- The image produced by the direct ophthalmoscope is the right way up and 15× magnified.

Eye drops should be applied in the following way:

FIRST WASH YOUR HANDS

i) Advise the patient to look up to the ceiling and away from the eye drop bottle

ii) Gently pull the lower eyelid down or ask the patient to do so; this will expose the lower fornix

iii) The bottle or Minims is placed directly above the exposed lower fornix, without touching it

iv) Apply the drop

v) Have a tissue ready to dab the cheek in case of over-spill but not touch the ocular surface

NB After some eyelid operations eye drops are applied **without** pulling the lid down. Instead the patient looks up and the drop is applied to the ocular surface medially

Figure 12.1

(a) Instilling eye drops

(b) Fluorescein staining of cornea—dendritic ulcer

(c) Using a Fluoret to apply fluorescein. With the lower lip pulled slightly downwards and away from the globe, the strip is gently placed in the conjunctival sac and the fluorescein released

(d) Inferior corneal abrasion staining with fluorescein

Fluorescein preparations

- Fluorescein paper strips (Fluorets)
- Single-dose fluorescein Minims
- Combined single-dose fluorescein with local anaesthetic, such as Minims proxymetacaine, is useful for measuring intraocular pressure by Goldmann tonometry

(a)
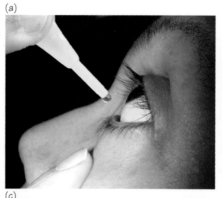

(b)
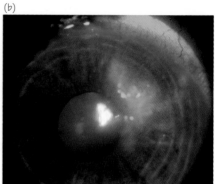

(c)
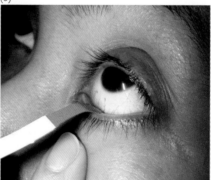

(d)
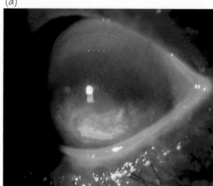

Figure 12.2 Dilating eye drops

Pupil size is controlled by the iris and its autonomic nervous innervation. The action of dilating drops is to modulate the effect of the autonomic control of the iris and ciliary body and hence pupil size

Accommodation of the lens (focusing ability) is controlled by the ciliary body which is also innervated by the parasympathetic nervous system and loss of this results in loss of accommodation (cycloplegia) with blurred near vision

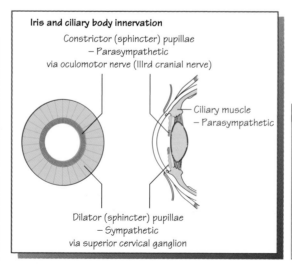

Iris and ciliary body innervation

Constrictor (sphincter) pupillae
– Parasympathetic
via oculomotor nerve (IIIrd cranial nerve)

Ciliary muscle
– Parasympathetic

Dilator (sphincter) pupillae
– Sympathetic
via superior cervical ganglion

DILATING DROPS WARNING!

► Warn patients of the after effects for the next few hours: i) blurred vision – especially for near vision and ii) glare in bright light

► Avoid driving until the effect has worn off

► Risk of precipitating an attack of *acute angle closure glaucoma* in patients with a narrow iridocorneal angle: the patient must see an ophthalmologist urgently if symptoms of blurred vision persist and a halo effect around a light source occurs

Ophthalmology at a Glance, Second Edition. Jane Olver, Lorraine Cassidy, Gurjeet Jutley, and Laura Crawley. © 2014 Jane Olver, Lorraine Cassidy, Gurjeet Jutley and Laura Crawley. Published 2014 by John Wiley & Sons, Ltd. Companion Website: www.ataglanceseries.com/ophthal

All eye examinations involve the insertion of eye drops, the most common being fluorescein, topical anaesthetic and dilating drops.

Aims
- Understand the indications for fluorescein, and the use of common dilating and anaesthetic drops.
- Know how to instil eye drops correctly (Figure 12.1).
- Be aware of the risks of dilating drops.

Definitions
- **Mydriatic**: drop that causes mydriasis (pupil dilation).
- **Miotic**: drop that causes miosis (pupil constriction).
- **Cycloplegia**: loss of accommodation caused by blocking the para-sympathetic innervation to the ciliary body.

Drops for ocular surface examination
Fluorescein
Fluorescein is an orange-brown crystalline substance and belongs to the triphenylmethane dyes. It is available as Minims drops or is dried onto paper (Fluoret). It adopts its characteristic yellow-green colour after dilution. Use a cobalt blue light from a slit lamp or direct ophthalmoscope to see the typical green-yellow fluorescence.
- Absorption spectrum: 465 and 490 nm (blue end).
- Emission spectrum: 520 and 530 nm (green-yellow region).

Fluorescein is water-soluble and does not stain the corneal epithelium (hydrophobic). It does stain the Bowman's membrane and stroma in an epithelial defect (e.g. dendritic ulcer).

> **TIP**
>
> Fluorescein stains soft contact lenses yellow-green; therefore, these should be removed prior to examination.

Rose Bengal
Rose Bengal is a red soluble dye and belongs to the group of fluorine dyes. It is available as a 1% Minims preparation. It stains wherever there is insufficient protection of the preocular tear film:
- Decreased tear components (e.g. keratoconjunctivitis sicca).
- Abnormal surface epithelial cells (e.g. degenerating or dead cells, or mucous strands).

Rose Bengal should be used very sparingly, as it causes stinging due to its acid properties. It is advisable to instil topical anaesthetic prior to its use and warn the patient about discomfort.

Topical anaesthetic drops
Topical anaesthesia is used:
- for ocular examination (tonometry and gonioscopy)
- for contact lens fitting
- to alleviate pain due to injury and to facilitate a thorough examination (e.g. for a foreign body, abrasion or ulcer)
- in children prior to instillation of often stingy eye drops.

These drops must be used sparingly and in short courses as they potentially mask the severity of pain if the injury worsens. Prolonged use is epithelial toxic.

Mode of action: they prevent generation and conduction of nerve impulses—and they mostly belong to the amine group of compounds.

Anaesthetic drops are obtainable in Minims without preservatives or in bottles with preservatives.

Oxybuprocaine 0.4% (Benoxinate)
Well absorbed with onset of action within 60 s. One drop lasts approximately 15 min.

Tetracaine 0.5% and 1.0% (Amethocaine)
Onset within 60 s, and effect lasts 20 min. Contact dermatitis has been reported.

Proxymetacaine 0.5% (Ophthaine)
Onset within 30 s, and the effect lasts 15 min. It is less stingy than the other anaesthetic drops listed here and is therefore useful in children. Also available as a combination with fluorescein in Minims, and is useful for Goldmann contact tonometry.

Common dilating drops for fundal examination
In order to examine the fundus adequately, the pupil needs to be dilated (Figure 12.2).

Tropicamide 1%
This is a synthetic analogue of atropine. It reduces the parasympathetic innervation to both the sphincter pupillae and the ciliary body, resulting in a marked mydriatic action and weak cycloplegic action. It is used alone or in combination with phenylephrine for better dilation.
- Maximum effect after 20–30 min.
- Effect wears off after at least 6 h.

Phenylephrine 2.5%
This is a synthetic compound and is biochemically closely related to adrenaline; it acts as a potent sympathomimetic. It stimulates dilator pupillae and causes mydriasis. However, the dilator pupillae is a weaker muscle than the sphincter pupillae, hence the mydriatic effect of phenylephrine is less than with tropicamide. It is used in combination with tropicamide or cyclopentolate. It is useful to help maximize dilation in dark brown irides.
- Maximum effect after 30 min.
- Effect wears off after 5 h.
- Phenylephrine 10% is rarely used due to systemic side effects.

Cyclopentolate 0.5% and 1%
This is a synthetic substance similar to atropine and has the advantage of being short acting and having a greater cycloplegic effect than tropicamide. It is commonly used in refraction in children to abolish accommodation.
- Mydriasis and cycloplegia within 20–30 min.
- Maximum cycloplegic effect lasts 45–60 min.
- Effect wears off after 24 h.

Side effects: risk of allergic reaction and raised intraocular pressure. In a baby <3 months old, cyclopentolate 0.5% should be used. Hypersensitivity is less common than with atropine. Rare side effects: visual hallucinations, disorientation and ataxia.

In patients with darkly pigmented irides, the cyclopentolate effect may be insufficient for full cycloplegia; therefore, use **atropine 1% drops**. Note that atropine has a longer acting period and a higher risk of side effects.

> **KEY POINTS**
>
> - Fluorescein needs a blue light to visualize its yellow colour.
> - Rose Bengal stains devitalized cells but should be used sparingly as it stings.
> - Tropicamide and cyclopentolate dilating drops also cause cycloplegia (blurring of near vision).
> - Proxymetacaine is the only topical anaesthetic that does not sting.

13 Red eye: the conjunctiva

Figure 13.1 Different types of red eye. (a) Acute anterior uveitis, (b) subjconjunctival haemorrhage, (c) drop toxicity causing red eyes and periocular skin and (d) viral conjunctivitis

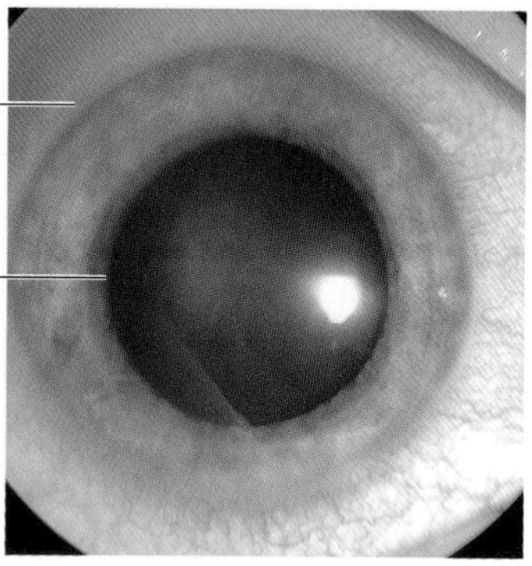

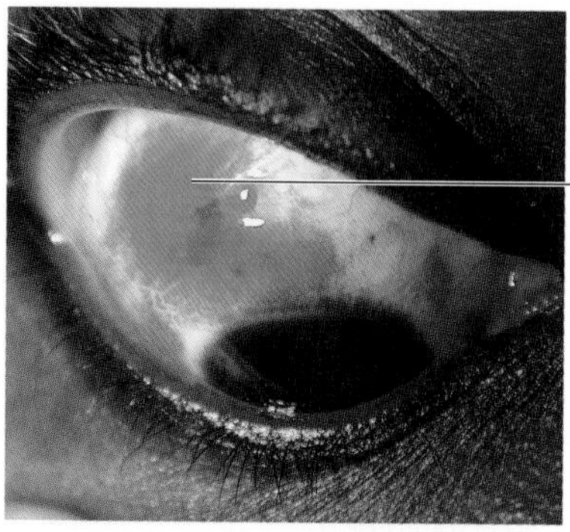

Note: See also Appendix 1: Red eye – signs and symptoms of different causes

(a)

Circumciliary injection
Pupil dilated by cycloplegic drops

(b)

Localized dense red haemorrhage

b) Subconjunctival haemorrhage – can be caused by trauma, hypertension or blood dyscrasia, but is most commonly idiopathic

(c)

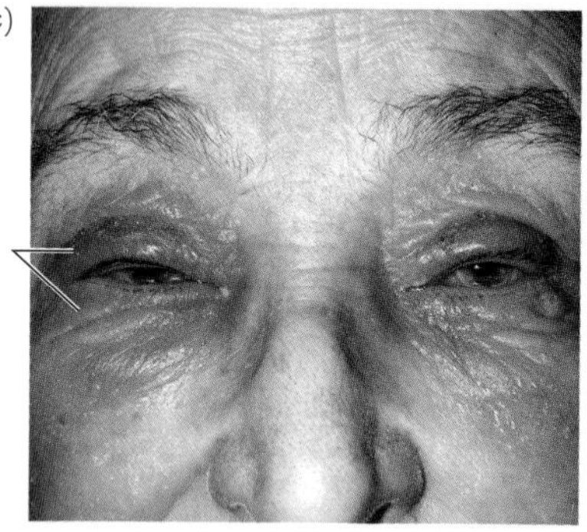

Periocular skin is red, dry and flaky

(d)

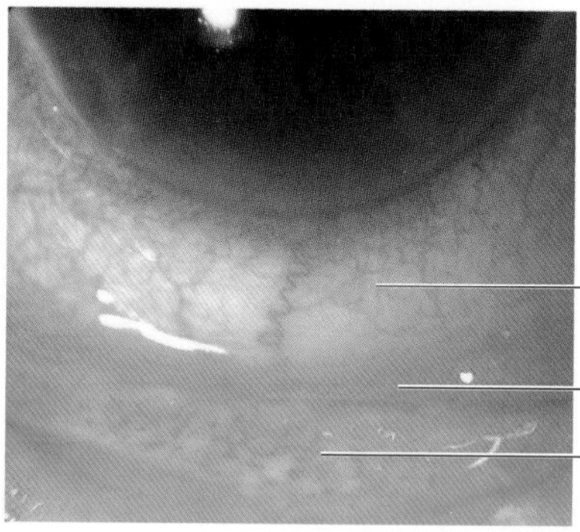

Generalized conjunctival redness
Tarsal conjunctival redness
Follicles

Figure 13.2 (a) Photographic and (b) schematic appearance of acute angle closure glaucoma – a sight threatening ophthalmic emergency

(a)

(b)

Fixed vertically oval pupil
Whorled iris appearance due to ischaemia
Brick red

WARNING

- Abnormal pupil shape or size
- Cloudy cornea
- Marked visual loss or photophobia
- Painful unilateral red eye with visual disturbance

Figure 13.3 Atopic conjunctivitis. Severe disease with corneal vascularization and perforation

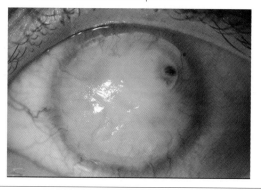

Figure 13.4 Stevens–Johnson syndrome. Corneal vascularization, scarring, cicatrical ectropian and dry ocular surface

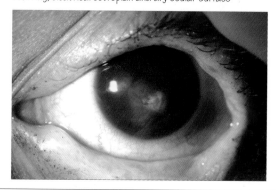

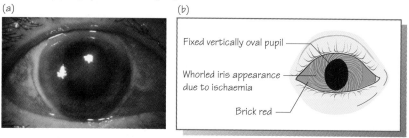

The red eye is a common complaint presenting to primary care and emergency eye clinics. Most do not have a sight-threatening cause; however, one must be alert to the 'red flag' signs to recognize those that do.

Aims of Chapters 13 and 14
- Identify the common causes of red eye (Figure 13.1).
- Recognize the sight-threatening causes of red eye.
- Understand when topical antibiotics and antivirals may be helpful.

Abnormal pupil shape
- A tear drop or misshapen pupil in the context of ocular trauma, however mild, is highly suggestive of penetrating ocular trauma or a severe blunt injury which has torn the pupil fibres or the iris root (insertion into the white sclera).
- A misshapen pupil in an acutely red eye without a history of ocular trauma suggests that posterior synechiae are present (the pupil is stuck to the lens behind.) This is highly suggestive of acute or recurrent inflammation as in anterior uveitis.
- A mid-dilated and fixed pupil in the context of a painful red eye is highly suggestive of acutely raised intraocular pressure (e.g. in acute glaucoma) (Figure 13.2).

Cloudy cornea
- You should be able to see the iris and pupil clearly through the cornea.
- There are many and varied causes of a cloudy cornea (infection as in contact lens ulcers, inflammation as in herpes-associated disciform keratitis, raised intraocular pressure, chemical injury etc.), and whilst it is not necessary to know why, you must seek expert ophthalmic advice promptly.

Marked visual loss or photophobia
- Photophobia is the predominant symptom in anterior uveitis and should be referred for an ophthalmic specialist opinion.

The conjunctiva
Infective conjunctivitis
Infective conjunctivitis is common and self-limiting in the majority of cases. Bacterial infections are more common in children (70–85%). Bacterial infections account for one-thirds to two-thirds of adult infections.
- *Symptoms*: red eye (usually bilateral), watering, discharge, itching or burning, crusting of the lid margins and general flu-like symptoms.
- *Signs*: diffuse redness across the conjunctiva and especially the tarsal conjunctiva (posterior surface of the lid); mucopurulent discharge.
- *Management*: hygiene advice (eye bathing and avoidance of towel sharing); topical antibiotics are not usually necessary as simple infective conjunctivitis is usually self-limiting, even in bacterial cases; topical lubricants will soothe and ease the itch; may take several weeks to resolve.

Special considerations
Chlamydial conjunctivitis
This is an oculogenital infection caused by serotypes D–K of *Chlamydia trachomatis*. It should be suspected in adults with a chronic non-resolving conjunctivitis with or without a history of venereal disease. Treatment with a tetracycline or azithromycin oral antibiotic is indicated, and patients should be referred to the genito-urinary medicine department for investigation and contact tracing.

Ophthalmia neonatorum (see Chapter 25)
Allergic conjunctivitis
Allergic conjunctivitis is common, affecting approximately 20% of the population, and it is commoner in atopic individuals. It may be acute and a type 1 hypersensitivity disorder, as in seasonal and perennial allergic conjunctivitis, or chronic with type 1 and 4 hypersensitivity reactions, as in vernal and atopic keratoconjunctivitis.

- *Symptoms*: itch (predominant symptom), watering.
- *Signs*: bilateral pink or red eyes, eyelid oedema, conjunctival swelling (chemosis) may be dramatic.

Refer to the table in Appendix 1 for more details on the signs and symptoms of different causes of red eye.

Subtypes
- *Seasonal allergic conjunctivitis (hay fever)*: allergens usually include tree and grass pollen; occurs in the spring and summer.
- *Perennial allergic conjunctivitis*: allergens include house dust mites and animal dander (skin scales); year-round symptoms.
- *Vernal allergic conjunctivitis*: primarily affects young boys in first decade of life; strong association with atopy; most cases remit by adulthood, with 5–10% persisting as atopic keratoconjunctivitis.
- *Atopic keratoconjunctivitis* (Figure 13.3): uncommon; chronic and unremitting; adults usually have a history of childhood atopy and vernal allergic conjunctivitis.

Giant papillary conjunctivitis
A response to mechanical trauma, this is traditionally induced by long-term soft contact lens wear but may occur in association with ocular prosthesis, filtering blebs created by glaucoma surgery and exposed sutures.

Management of allergic eye disease
- Mast cell stabilizers.
- Antihistamines (oral and topical).
- Topical steroids may be indicated in severe cases, but ophthalmic advice should be sought.
- Vernal and atopic keratoconjunctivitis require specialist ophthalmic care. Some patients require systemic immunosuppression.

Stevens–Johnson syndrome (Figure 13.4)
- Uncommon potentially lethal condition with severe ocular morbidity.
- Type IV hypersensitivity reaction.
- Triggers include infections (mycoplasma, HSV, mycobacteria, Grp A streptococci, and others), drugs (sulphonamides, barbiturates, penicillins, anti-epileptics and antiretrovirals), malignancy and idiopathic.
- Acute disease usually associated with crusty lids and a transient self-limiting conjunctivitis. Membranes may form on the inner surface of the lids.
- Late disease is associated with marked dry eye as the goblet cells and lacrimal gland ductules are destroyed. This may lead to breakdown of the corneal and ocular surface, scarring, symblepharon formation (permanent adhesion of the conjunctiva in the depths of fornices of the lids to the globe), aberrant and misdirected lashes, entropian and corneal stem cell failure causing blindness.

Subconjunctival haemorrhage
- Painless localized dense red haemorrhage on the surface of an otherwise normal eye.
- Common and self-limiting (resolves in 10–14 days).
- Sudden onset and often incidental finding.
- Some evidence indicates that it is more common in systemic hypertension.
- Routine investigation for coagulopathies is not indicated unless there is evidence and clinical suspicion of other bleeding sites.

KEY POINTS

- Red flags in a patient with red eye: abnormal pupil shape or size, cloudy cornea, marked visual loss or photophobia, and painful unilateral red eye with acute visual disturbance.
- Simple conjunctivitis is usually unpleasant but self-limiting.

Figure 14.1 (a) Linear and (b) large corneal abrasions

(a)
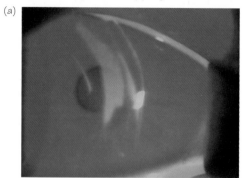

(b)
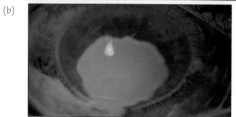

Figure 14.2 Corneal foreign bodies

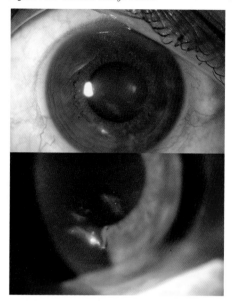

Figure 14.3 Pseudomonas keratitis: contact lens ulcer with hypopyon (white cells in the anterior chamber settled inferiorly)

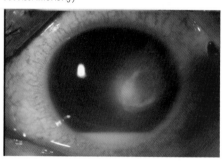

Figure 14.4 Acanthoemeba keratitis: (a) ring abscess and (b) perineural infiltrates

(a)
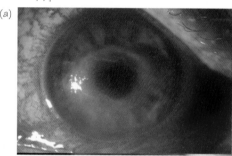

(b)
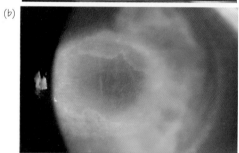

Figure 14.5 Dendritic ulcer

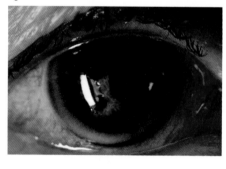

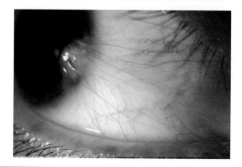

Figure 14.6 Pterygium

Ophthalmology at a Glance, Second Edition. Jane Olver, Lorraine Cassidy, Gurjeet Jutley, and Laura Crawley. © 2014 Jane Olver, Lorraine Cassidy, Gurjeet Jutley and Laura Crawley. Published 2014 by John Wiley & Sons, Ltd. Companion Website: www.ataglanceseries.com/ophthal

A complete examination of a red eye involves instilling fluorescein drops either in 2% form or mixed with a local anaesthetic drop such as proxymetacaine and illuminating the ocular surface with cobalt blue light. This allows you to see pathology not visible under white light, namely, disruption of the corneal surface including abrasions, ulceration and corneal and conjunctival epithelial disturbance.

> **Golden rule**
>
> • **Never** prescribe topical steroids to a patient with a fluorescein staining of the cornea.
> Steroid eye drops significantly exacerbate herpetic dendritic corneal ulcers. They have a role in managing the inflammatory component of corneal infections; initiation of topical steroid drops should be undertaken only by an ophthalmologist.

Corneal abrasions (Figure 14.1)

• Corneal abrasions (scratches) occur when the surface layer of the corneal epithelium is disturbed, usually by trauma (e.g. finger poking, or a tree branch or bamboo stake in the eye).
• Corneal abrasions are extremely painful but usually resolve after 48 h.
• Fluorescein staining reveals an epithelial defect under cobalt blue light.
• Upper lid eversion and careful examination of the upper and lower fornices are advised to look for retained foreign bodies (Figure 14.2).
• Topical chloramphenicol drops or ointment is usually prescribed. An eye pad is not necessary. Topical anaesthetic to take away is **contraindicated**.
• In severe cases, the patient may develop recurrent corneal erosion syndrome where the new corneal epithelium re-opens or sloughs off repeatedly, causing recurrent pain, foreign body sensation and mildly blurred vision. These cases should be referred for specialist management. The aetiology is often a sharp injury from a baby's fingernail, sharp-leafed plant or edge of paper. An underlying corneal dystrophy is a rare underlying cause.

Corneal infections

• Serious corneal infections are usually seen in contact lens wearers, in farmers or gardeners where unusual organisms such as fungi or *Acanthamoeba* should be suspected, in cases of herpes simplex or zoster and in patients where there is disruption to normal corneal innervation causing reduced or absent corneal sensation.

Contact lens keratitis (Figure 14.3)

• A unilateral painful red eye in a contact lens wearer is highly suspicious for a contact lens ulcer or keratitis.
• Some bacterial pathogens are aggressive and can cause corneal perforation (e.g. *Pseudomonas aeruginosa*).

Symptoms
• Unilateral red eye.
• Pain and photophobia.
• Tearing.
• Contact lens over-wear or unintentional overnight wear.

Signs
• Unilateral red eye.
• You may see a white spot on the cornea with the naked eye.
• Fluorescein staining reveals an epithelial defect under cobalt blue light.

Management
• Urgent ophthalmic opinion.
• Corneal scrape for urgent Gram staining; microscopy and culture for bacteria, fungi and *Acanthamoeba*.

• Contact lens wear break.
• Frequent topical antibiotics, usually a quinolone such as ofloxacin or levofloxacin.

Acanthamoeba keratitis (Figure 14.4)

• *Acanthamoeba* spp. are found in soil, fresh or brackish water and the upper respiratory tract.
• *A. keratitis* causes serious corneal infections in contact lens wearers (especially if they rinse their lenses in tap water) and in agricultural workers who sustain soil-contaminated corneal injuries.
• *A. keratitis* should be suspected in one of these at-risk groups where the pain and visual disturbance are out of keeping with the clinical signs.
• Classical signs include ring infiltrates and perineural infiltrates.
• Special culture media such as an *Escherichia coli*-seeded non-nutrient agar plate are required to grow the organism, or the amoebic cysts can be seen in the cornea with laser confocal microscopy.
• Treatment is continued for months as viable organisms can encyst and lie dormant in the cornea only to reactivate in the future.
• Topical amoebicides include propramidine isethionate 0.1% (Brolene), polyhexamethylene biguanide 0.02% drops, hexamindine and chlorhexidine.

Dendritic ulcers (Figure 14.5)

• Herpes simplex virus (HSV) detection by polymerase chain reaction in the trigeminal ganglion is almost 100% in people over the age of 60, yet only 20–25% of individuals with HSV antibodies have a clinical history of the disease.
• HSV can cause a characteristic branching tree-like ulcer on the cornea known as a dendritic ulcer.
• HSV lies dormant in the trigeminal ganglion but can be reactivated to cause recurrent corneal ulceration.
• In the longer term, the corneal sensation may be reduced or absent, and this is associated with long-term scarring, melting, vascularization and failure of the cornea.
• Corneal sensation should be checked and compared with the fellow eye before fluorescein and topical anaesthetic drops are instilled.

Management
• Topical acyclovir 3% ointment five times daily.
• Alternatives include trifluorothymidine, vidarabine and ganciclovir.

Pterygium (Figure 14.6)

• A pterygium is a triangular or wedge-shaped growth of conjunctival tissue onto the cornea.
• It is thought to be more common in individuals with high ultraviolet light exposure.
• In most cases it does not interfere with vision, but where it encroaches on the central vision or distorts the shape of the eye, causing astigmatism, it can be treated surgically.
• It may become inflamed periodically, and topical lubricants or nonsteroidal or steroid drops may be necessary.

> **KEY POINTS**
>
> • Initiation of topical steroid drops should be undertaken only by an ophthalmologist.
> • A unilateral painful red eye in a contact lens wearer is highly suspicious for a contact lens ulcer or keratitis and should be referred urgently.

Figure 15.1 Episcleritis. Benign localized inflammation of the episclera (a)– the layer lying beneath the conjunctiva and superficial to the sclera (b). Usually idiopathic but may be associated with a rheumatological disorder. No symptoms or mild dull pain. No treatment required. If severe pain, suspect **scleritis,** which is more serious and needs investigating

(a)

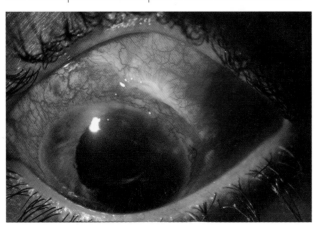

(b)

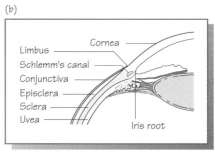

Limbus —
Schlemm's canal —
Conjunctiva —
Episclera —
Sclera —
Uvea —
Cornea —
Iris root —

Figure 15.2 Scleritis. This is a case of necrotizing scleritis in a patient with congenital glaucoma. Note the widespread redness and patch of scleral necrosis at 11 o'clock

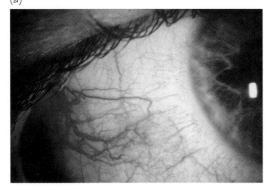

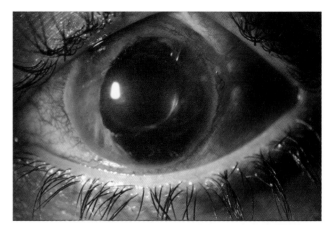

Figure 15.3 Marked scleromalacia. The white sclera has melted and the uveal tissue is seen prolapsing through, covered by only a thin layer of conjunctiva

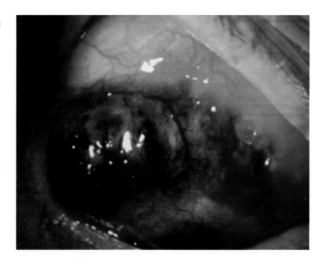

Ophthalmology at a Glance, Second Edition. Jane Olver, Lorraine Cassidy, Gurjeet Jutley, and Laura Crawley. © 2014 Jane Olver, Lorraine Cassidy, Gurjeet Jutley and Laura Crawley. Published 2014 by John Wiley & Sons, Ltd. Companion Website: www.ataglanceseries.com/ophthal

The wall of the globe consists of three main layers:
• Conjunctiva: the outer transparent mucous membrane of the globe. It also lines the inner surface of the lids and forms the depths or fornices of the lids. The conjunctiva contains blood vessels, lymphatics, mucus producing goblet cells, accessory lacrimal glands (glands of Krause and Wolfring) and lymphoid tissue (see also Chapter 13).
• Episclera: a middle layer of connective tissue and blood vessels.
• Sclera: the white inner coat of the eye. It is composed of collagen bundles.

Episcleritis (Figure 15.1a)

This is a common, benign and recurrent condition where the episcleral tissue becomes inflamed. It is usually idiopathic and self-limiting, although speed of resolution can be enhanced with topical or oral anti-inflammatories.

Presentation

Commonly unilateral, but there may be bilateral, sectorial redness of the eye. It is usually seen in the temporal or nasal quadrants of the eye, but may occasionally be diffuse through 360°. It is uncomfortable but not very painful. When a patient has severe pain, scleritis is more likely.

Treatment

Very mild episcleritis may not require any treatment.
• Lubricants.
• Topical non-steroidal anti-inflammatory drugs (NSAIDs) (e.g. ketorolac 3× daily).
• Oral NSAIDs (check for contraindications) ibuprofen, flurbiprofen or diclofenac.
• Topical mild steroids (e.g. prednisolone 0.3% or 0.5% 3× daily for 10–14 days).

Scleritis (Figure 15.2)

Scleritis is much less common than episcleritis. It may be mild and self-limiting or severe, extremely painful and sight threatening (see Chapter 19).

It is commonly classified into anterior and posterior disease and as necrotizing or non-necrotizing.

There is an associated systemic condition in 33–50% of scleritis, such as:
• rheumatoid arthritis
• systemic vasculitides
• Wegener's granulomatosis, more recently renamed granulomatosis with polyangiitis
• systemic lupus erythematosis
• seronegative spondyloarthropathies.
It is also associated with infection, especially tuberculosis and syphilis; trauma, including surgical trauma; and malignancy, such as lymphoma.

Signs

• Intense redness of the scleral and episcleral vessels.
• Tender globe to touch.
• Scleral necrosis in necrotizing disease, scleromalacia, see Figure 15.3. The black-blue hue of the choroidal tissue is seen as the white scleral tissue disintegrates.

Management

The traditional treatment algorithm involves:
• NSAIDS.
• Local depot steroid injections (e.g. orbital floor or subconjunctival steroid).
• Oral steroids 1–2 mg/kg/day.
• Cytotoxic agents (e.g. cyclophosphamide, methotrexate and azathioprine).
• Biologic agents (e.g. anti-CD20 (Rituximab)).
In addition:
• Seek out and manage associated systemic conditions.
• Systemic immunosuppression is often required.
• Specialist management is required in most cases.

KEY POINTS

• Episcleritis is usually sectorial, is associated with a low pain score and responds to topical NSAIDs.
• Scleritis is typically very painful and requires specialist management.

---

16 Ophthalmic trauma principles and management of chemical injuries

Ophthalmic trauma

1. Chemical: EMERGENCY
2. Blunt (Chapter 16)
3. Sharp and penetrating (Chapter 16)

The principles of eye trauma

These are as any trauma:
A. Primary survey and Resuscitation
   1. Airway
   2. Breathing
   3. C-spine
   4. Cardiovascular
B. Secondary survey. Look, listen, feel!
   Top to toe, includes orbits and eyes

Medicolegal considerations

All trauma cases should be regarded as potential medicolegal cases especially when an alleged assault has taken place or there is an occupational injury. Take a meticulous history, record the best visual acuity, do a very careful clinical examination, record your findings clearly in the notes. Always sign and print your name, plus date the entry giving the time that you examined the patient

Figure 16.1 Parts of the eye and orbit that can be commonly involved in trauma

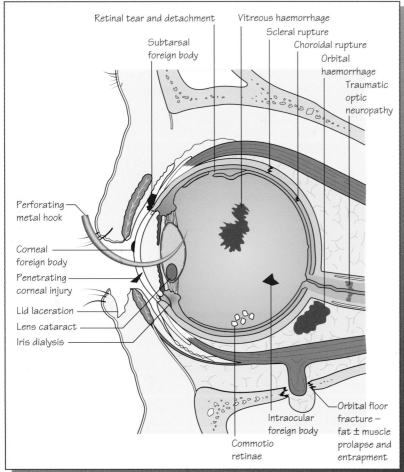

Retinal tear and detachment
Vitreous haemorrhage
Subtarsal foreign body
Scleral rupture
Choroidal rupture
Orbital haemorrhage
Traumatic optic neuropathy
Perforating metal hook
Corneal foreign body
Penetrating corneal injury
Lid laceration
Lens cataract
Iris dialysis
Intraocular foreign body
Commotio retinae
Orbital floor fracture – fat ± muscle prolapse and entrapment

Examination

- Take a thorough history and record exactly what happened
- Measure the visual acuity (in chemical injury can do after washout)
- Examine the eye systematically from the outside lids to the retina, including pupil reactions
- **Dilate pupils for fundal examination**
- ± Radiological investigation
- Photograph for medicolegal purposes

Figure 16.2 How to wash out a chemical injury

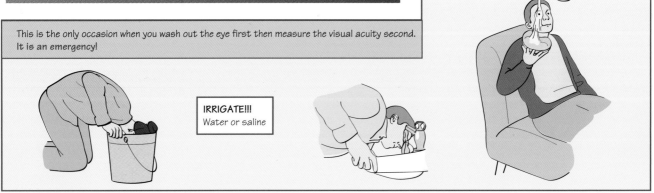

This is the only occasion when you wash out the eye first then measure the visual acuity second. It is an emergency!

IRRIGATE!!!
Water or saline

Ophthalmology at a Glance, Second Edition. Jane Olver, Lorraine Cassidy, Gurjeet Jutley, and Laura Crawley. © 2014 Jane Olver, Lorraine Cassidy, Gurjeet Jutley and Laura Crawley. Published 2014 by John Wiley & Sons, Ltd. Companion Website: www.ataglanceseries.com/ophthal

Managing simple eye trauma is a basic requirement for a casualty officer. Knowing how to manage more complex trauma requires you to identify the extent of the eye trauma, stabilize it and know when and to whom to refer the patient.

Aims

- List the main causes of loss of vision due to trauma.
- Know how to wash out a chemical injury.

Principles of ophthalmic trauma

The ophthalmic trauma patient may be managed by the ophthalmologist alone or by the ophthalmologist working in a team with the plastic, maxillofacial or neurosurgeon, if there are associated severe facial and head injuries.

The five main causes of loss of vision with trauma are:

1 Corneal scarring and anterior segment damage from severe alkali burn
2 Severe disrupted globe from a penetrating injury (e.g. road traffic accident)
3 Unrecognized intraocular metallic foreign body causing siderosis bulbi
4 Compressive optic neuropathy from retrobulbar haemorrhage
5 Traumatic optic neuropathy from optic canal bony or shearing injury.

Trauma can affect the periocular region, bony orbit, orbital contents, globe or optic nerve (Figure 16.1).
- **Eyelid and periocular and orbital haematoma**—fully assess to rule out orbital floor fracture and fracture of base of skull.
- **Orbital bony wall fracture**—floor > medial wall with diplopia; needs repair.
- **Eyelid subtarsal foreign body**—evert lid and remove with cotton bud.
- **Eyelids**—partial or full thickness laceration: explore wound, exclude penetrating eye injury and repair within 48 h.
- **Lacrimal drainage system**—most commonly lower canaliculus; needs oculoplastics repair and stent (e.g. MiniMonaka tube).
- **Conjunctival laceration**—may need suturing; exclude more extensive deeper injury.
- **Corneal abrasion**—treat with topical antibiotics ± cycloplegia and an eye pad.
- **Corneal foreign body**—needs removal and dilated fundoscopy.
- **Corneal penetrating injury ± sclera, iris, lens or retinal injury**—all require urgent surgical repair.
- **Hypahaema (blood in the anterior chamber)**—can cause secondary glaucoma; needs urgent ophthalmic assessment.
- **Dislocated lens**—may need surgery to remove lens.
- **Traumatic cataract**—most need surgical removal.
- **Glaucoma secondary to angle recession (i.e. damage to trabecular meshwork)**—needs specialist treatment.
- **Blunt vitreous haemorrhage and retinal commotio**—needs vitreo-retinal assessment to exclude retinal tear.
- **Retinal tear or dialysis**—needs urgent retinal surgery.

- **Choroidal rupture**—may lose vision if it underlies the macula; untreatable.
- **Scleral perforation**—needs surgical exploration and repair; if extensive, patient may lose eye (enucleation).
- **Massive retrobulbar haemorrhage**—needs urgent lateral canthotomy or cantholysis to decompress orbit.
- **Traumatic optic neuropathy**—needs to be treated with high-dose steroids within hours.
- **Traumatic cranial nerve injury**—IVth, IIIrd and VIth cranial nerves need magnetic resonance imaging scan.
- **Complete globe disruption**—needs enucleation within 14 days to prevent sympathetic ophthalmia.

If any of the above are suspected, refer *immediately* to eye casualty.

Chemical injuries (Figure 16.2)

Which chemical? Substances include alkalis (lime, cement, plaster or ammonia), acids, solvents, detergents, irritants (e.g. mace and pepper) and super glue. Alkalis (e.g. ammonia or wet cement) are the most destructive, penetrating the deep layers of the eye with time. In high concentrations, they cause severe ischaemia of the conjunctiva, corneal limbus, cornea and sclera, and cause subsequent scarring and blindness. There may be associated severe uveitis and cataract formation.

How to manage a patient with a suspected chemical eye injury

1 **Wash out the eye immediately.**
2 Measure the pH of the tear meniscus if litmus paper is handy.
3 Otherwise, apply immediately topical anaesthetic drops if handy.
4 Copious irrigation with normal saline or Ringer's solution. If neither is available, put the patient's head under a cold water tap or into a bowl of cold water—with the eyes open! Irrigate or splash the eyes for 5–10 min, then repeat the pH measurement.
5 Ensure that the surface of the eye and the upper and lower fornices are included. Using a cotton bud, evert the upper lid, check for fragments of cement and the like and remove them. Swipe the cotton bud along the lower fornix to remove particulate debris.
6 Now measure the visual acuity and check the eye, including the intraocular pressure (IOP).
7 Admit.
8 Topical treatment: intensive topical antibiotics, vitamin C and cycloplegia (to prevent pain) ± steroids. Treat raised IOP as necessary.
9 Oral high-dose vitamin C.
10 Later surgery if needed—limbal cell transplant and penetrating keratoplasty (corneal graft).

KEY POINTS

- All trauma cases are medico-legal cases until proved otherwise.
- Ocular trauma can result from a chemical, blunt or sharp (penetrating) injury.
- Alkali burns can cause blindness and must be irrigated immediately.

---

17 Specific features of blunt and sharp injuries

Blunt injuries

Figure 17.1 Acute massive orbital haemorrhage with proptosis. Note: may need urgent lateral cantholysis and canthotomy to drain a traumatic retrobulbar haemorrhage

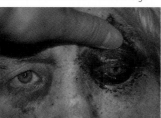

Figure 17.2 Subconjunctival haemorrhage and chemosis

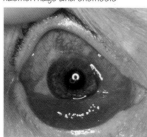

Figure 17.3 Hyphaema

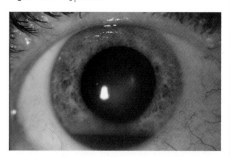

Figure 17.4 Dislocated lens

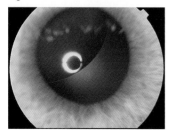

Figure 17.5 CT scan of left orbital medial wall and floor fracture – patient has severe left enophthalmos and diplopia from restricted eye movement

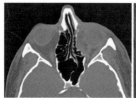
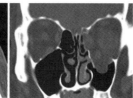

Figure 17.6 Bungee cord choroidal rupture

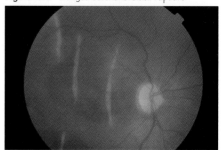

Sharp injuries

WARNING

▶ Exclude small entry wound of an intraocular foreign body (IOFB). Dilate the pupil and examine the fundus to exclude IOFB. If there is a history of hammering, use orbital X-ray or CT to exclude IOFB

Figure 17.7 Corneal perforation with fishing hook – may have perforated lens

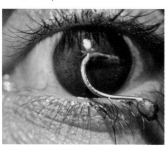

Figure 17.8 Intraocular foreign body. Needs vitrectomy and removal

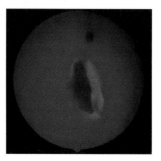

Figure 17.9 Medial eyelid and lacrimal canaliculus avulsion. Needs primary repair and canalicular intubation

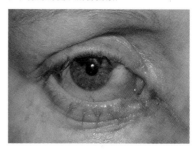

Figure 17.10 (a) and (b) Corneal foreign bodies. These need to be removed with a cotton bud or sharp needle with good illumination and magnification. May leave a rust ring which needs later further removal with a needle

(a)
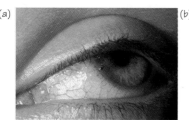
(b)
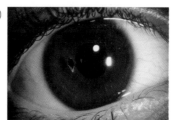

Figure 17.11 Corneal abrasion

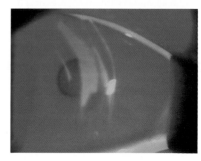

Ophthalmology at a Glance, Second Edition. Jane Olver, Lorraine Cassidy, Gurjeet Jutley, and Laura Crawley. © 2014 Jane Olver, Lorraine Cassidy, Gurjeet Jutley and Laura Crawley. Published 2014 by John Wiley & Sons, Ltd. Companion Website: www.ataglanceseries.com/ophthal

Aims
• Know how to manage a retrobulbar haemorrhage; remove a corneal foreign body (FB); and manage a corneal abrasion.

Blunt injuries
Aetiology
From a fist; cricket, squash or tennis ball; champagne cork or the like.
Findings
Lid ecchymosis, orbital (Figure 17.1) and subconjunctival (Figure 17.2) haemorrhage, hyphaema (Figure 17.3), lens injury (Figure 17.4), orbital floor fracture (Figure 17.5), vitreous haemorrhage and commotion retinae (Figure 17.6).
Systematic examination
Front (eyelids) to the back (retina) including the orbit. Exclude a perforating ocular injury. Exclude an orbital floor fracture by examining the eye movements, particularly restriction of upgaze, and look for infra-orbital numbness. Examine the cornea and conjunctiva for FBs abrasions and lacerations. Use fluorescein drops to visualize corneal abrasions. Examine the fundus.
Blunt injury: traumatic hyphaema
Blood in the anterior chamber. Often microscopic and only detected on the slit lamp or forms a fluid level easily seen with a pen torch. If blood fills the entire anterior chamber—'blackball hyphaema'.
Management: If the posterior segment of the eye cannot be seen easily, do an ultrasound for vitreous, supra- or sub-retinal haemorrhage; Steroid and dilating drops minimize inflammation and re-bleeding. Surgical washout of blood is rarely required except in blackball hyphaema with intractably raised intraocular pressure.
Traumatic iritis
Inflammation in the anterior chamber (AC) of the eye seen as white cells and flare on the slit lamp. Common even after minor blunt trauma to the globe causing symptoms of pain, photophobia and blurred vision.
Management: Treat with topical steroid and mydriatic drops.
Orbital haematoma
Eyelid ecchymosis. Test consensual pupillary reflex by shining a bright light through the bruised lid to confirm that the afferent pathway is working. With established eyelid bruising, it is difficult to open the eyelids and examine without using topical anaesthesia and fingers to prise open the lids. Measure the visual acuity, examine the eye movements, exclude a perforating injury and look at the fundus.

Retrobulbar haemorrhage—Emergency

This is an ophthalmic emergency and can cause rapid blindness. Compartment syndrome within the orbit causes pain, proptosis, reduced vision and poor pupil reactions. It occurs following periocular anaesthesia or blunt trauma and can be associated with a carotico-cavernous fistula.
Management:
Emergency lateral canthotomy and cantholysis to relieve high orbital pressure and reduce the risk of compressive optic neuropathy.

Commotio retinae (CR) or 'retinal bruising'
The retina is opaque. If the central retina or macula is affected, the vision can be blurred. CR usually resolves fully.
Traumatic optic neuropathy
Associated with severe head trauma and multiple injuries. Prognosis for visual recovery is poor when a marked afferent pupillary defect.
Management: Conservative. High-dose intravenous steroids have not demonstrated significant benefit for visual recovery.
Orbital floor fracture
Blow-out fracture of the floor or medial wall into the sinus. Orbital tissue entrapment may cause diplopia and limited eye movements. Enophthalmic often after swelling has settled.
Management: If there is painful restriction of upgaze, do urgent orbital floor repair. If there are persistent restrictive eye movements or enophthalmos after one week, do orbital floor repair.

Sharp, penetrating and perforating injuries
Aetiology (Figure 17.7)
Sharp objects (e.g. glass, spiky plants, hammer and chisel, or fish hooks) cause eyelid, corneoscleral, iris, lens and retinal lacerations.
Findings (Figure 17.8 and Figure 17.9)
The entry wound may be tiny and a high index of suspicion is required in all high-velocity injuries for the presence of an interocular FB (IOFB). Misshapen pupils suggest penetrating injury. Perforating injuries require urgent exploration under general anaesthesia to assess the full extent of the injury and to do the micro-surgical repair.
Superficial corneal injuries (Figure 17.10)
Corneal FBs and subtarsal FBs (STFBs) are common. The patient often gives a history of dust, metal or an insect entering the eye.
Symptoms: Painful photophobic red watering eye, sensation of FB on eye or under eyelid, often completely relieved on the instillation of topical local anaesthetic.
Signs: Corneal FB on the corneal epithelium seen with a pen torch or slit lamp; STFBs are found on the tarsal conjunctiva when the upper lid is everted, and they typically cause repeated vertical streak corneal abrasions with repeated blinking.
Corneal abrasion (Figure 17.10)
History of scratch from a sharp plant, paper, fingernail or the like.
Symptoms: Severe pain and FB sensation, photophobia and watering.
Signs: Red eye, fluorescein staining of the epithelial defect in cobalt blue light. Corneal abrasions are very painful but heal quickly. When from a very sharp object, recurrent erosion syndrome (RES) can develop where the new epithelial cells do not adhere well to the underlying stroma and repeatedly slough off. This is treated with lubricating drops and ointment before sleeping.
Examination: Topical anaesthesia and fluorescein to demonstrate a corneal abrasion; In all cases, the upper lid must be everted (see Chapter 10) to look for a retained STFB.
Management: Wipe off the corneal or subtarsal FB with a cotton bud, or tip of an orange needle to scrape or flick the FB off; Prescribe topical chloramphenicol drops 4× daily for 5 days. A pad is not necessary. With marked pain and photophobia, cyclopentolate 1% may be used 3× daily. Do not prescribe topical anaesthesia to take home.
Corneal laceration
A corneal laceration can be self sealing but usually requires microscopic suturing and exploration.

KEY POINTS
• Retrobulbar haemorrhage—lateral canthotomy and cantholysis saves vision.
• Evert the upper lid to detect and remove a subtarsal FB.
• Corneal abrasion caused by a sharp object may cause RES.

Figure 18.1 The non-inflamed eye

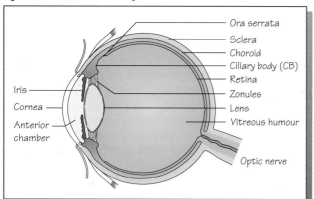

Ora serrata
Sclera
Choroid
Ciliary body (CB)
Retina
Zonules
Lens
Vitreous humour

Iris
Cornea
Anterior chamber

Optic nerve

Figure 18.2 Changes in the eye caused by inflammation

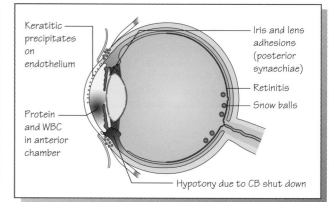

Keratitic precipitates on endothelium

Protein and WBC in anterior chamber

Iris and lens adhesions (posterior synaechiae)
Retinitis
Snow balls

Hypotony due to CB shut down

Figure 18.3 Uveitis

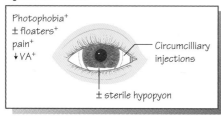

Photophobia⁺
± floaters⁺
pain⁺
↓VA⁺

Circumcilliary injections

± sterile hypopyon

Figure 18.4 Anterior uveitis with granulomatous keratoprecipitates

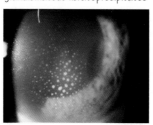

Figure 18.5 Scleritis

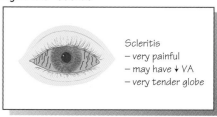

Scleritis
– very painful
– may have ↓ VA
– very tender globe

The underlying causes and management of uveitis

Consider infective aetiology?
- Is this VIRAL?
  - Examples include HSV, CMV, HZV and EBV
- Is this BACTERIAL?
  - Examples include Tuberculosis, *Borrelia burgdorferi* and syphilis
- Is this FUNGAL?
  - Examples include *Candida, Aspergillus* and histoplasmosis
- Is this PROTOZOAN?
  - Examples include *Toxoplasma gondii* and *Toxocara canis*

Consider non-infective aetiology?
- Is this GRANULOMATOUS?
  - Examples include Sarcoidosis, Wegener's and vasculitides
- Is this NON-GRANULOMATOUS?
  - If yes, is this seropositive?
    - Examples include rheumatoid arthritis, Sjogren's syndrome and polyarteritis nodosa
    - These are a slightly unusual set of disorders as they don't affect the uveal tract per se but, rather, cause inflammation of the sclera
    - One exception is juvenile idiopathic arthritis, which causes a painless acute anterior uveitis
  - Or is this seronegative?
    - Examples include HLA-B27 diseases, such as ankylosing spondylitis (exclusively seen in anterior uveitis) and Behçet's disease

Table 18.1 Uveitis can lead to loss of vision

Complication	Mechanism
Posterior synaechiae	Iris and lens adhesions make it increasingly difficult for aqueous to leave the pupil into the trabeculum. The buildup of pressure in the posterior chamber causes the iris to bow forward and thus compromise the angle further, a so-called iris bombe
Glaucoma	Multi-factorial, including: • Clogging up of trabecular meshwork from inflammatory cells • Iris bombe (so called 'pupil block') • 20% of the population have increased pressure due to steroids (steroid-responders)
Hypotony	Inflammation and shutdown of the ciliary body
Band keratopathy	Chronic inflammation alters the pH of the ocular surface, favoring the precipitation of calcium salts
Cataract	May be primary or secondary to systemic steroids of long-term topical steroid drops
Cystoid macula oedema	Inflammation disturbs the blood–retinal barrier

KEY POINTS

- Anterior uveitis is very common in the emergency department
- Posterior uveitis can cause loss of vision
- Posterior scleritis inflammation is very painful

Ophthalmology at a Glance, Second Edition. Jane Olver, Lorraine Cassidy, Gurjeet Jutley, and Laura Crawley. © 2014 Jane Olver, Lorraine Cassidy, Gurjeet Jutley and Laura Crawley. Published 2014 by John Wiley & Sons, Ltd. Companion Website: www.ataglanceseries.com/ophthal

Uveitis (Figures 18.1, 18.2 and 18.3) is inflammation of the uveal tract and can be anterior (Figure 18.4), intermediate or posterior. It can give blurred vision and lead to loss of vision (Table 18.1).

Aims

1 Characterize and diagnose the types of uveitis.
2 Know the most common causes of inflammation in the eye affecting the vision (e.g. scleritis).

We classify ocular inflammation anatomically: for instance, anterior uveitis is inflammation of the iris, retinitis is inflammation of the retina, scleritis is inflammation of the sclera (Figure 18.5) and episcleritis is inflammation of the episclera.

Uveitis

- Acute anterior uveitis (AAU): inflammation of the iris and ciliary body.
  - *Symptoms:* Acute onset pain, photophobia and secondary watering. **Exception**: juvenile idiopathic arthropathy (JIA) anterior uveitis is **painless**.
  - *Signs:* Red eye with conjunctival circumciliary injection (around the limbus; Figure 18.3), kerato precipitates (white blood cells (WBC) on the corneal endothelium; Figure 18.4), posterior synechiae (inflammatory cells causing adhesions between the lens and iris) and cells and flare in the anterior chamber (corresponding to WBC and proteins following the breakdown of the blood–iris barrier); seen on the slit lamp.
- Intermediate uveitis: inflammatory signs in the vitreous
  - *Symptoms:* floaters, blurred vision, without pain.
  - *Signs:* vitreous cells, snowballs (pre-retinal inflammatory aggregates), snow-banking (pars plana exudation), and macular oedema.
- Posterior uveitis
  - Can be a chorioretinitis, affecting both the chorid (uvea) and the adjacent retina.
  - *Symptoms:* Painless blurring of vision, with floaters and photopsia (flashing light).
  - *Signs:* variable cells in the anterior chamber and vitreous, choroiditis (fluffy, raised lesions without pigment if active), retinitis (cotton wool spots, haemorrhages and cuffing, attenuation or dilatation of vessels), macular oedema and exudative retinal detachment.
  - Specific inflammatory disorders that target the choroidal tissue are known as the white dot syndromes.
- Pan-uveitis: affecting all the above, anterior, intermediate and posterior.

Investigations

Distinguish whether the uveitis is infective or non-infective. Sixty percent of uveitis is idiopathic, with important underlying systemic disease in the remainder.

Do baseline and specific tests: full blood count (FBC); urea and electrolytes (U&E); chest X-ray (CXR); angiotensin-converting enzyme (ACE); human leukocyte antigen tests (HLA-B27 and HLA-A29); syphilis (Venereal Disease Research Laboratory (VDRL) test); enzyme-linked immunosorbent spot (ELISPOT) assay; lyme serology; antinuclear antibody (ANA) test and anti-neutrophil cytoplasmic antibodies (ANCA) test.

Management

All idiopathic causes of uveitis are treated as non-infective.

Infective

- If the cause of the inflammation is infective, the most appropriate antimicrobial should be used.

- Note the Jarisch–Herxheimer reaction, an inflammatory reaction against massive bacterial lysis once antimicrobials commence, particularly with syphilis and tuberculosis, which can be reduced with corticosteroids added to the antimicrobials.

Non-infectious

- Corticosteroids applied topically, peri-ocularly, orally or intravenously. Liaise with the physicians to help control patients' uveitis with steroid- sparing agents.
- Advances in nanotechnology of sustained-release implants placed directly in the vitreous deliver local steroid to the back of the eye, thus negating problems of poor safety profile and reduced bioavailability of oral steroids due to the blood–retinal barrier (choriocapillaris).

Posterior scleritis

- *Symptoms:* anterior scleritis (diffuse, nodular or necrotising) has typical deep injection (redness) and pain. In posterior scleritis, the eye is often white but the posterior sclera is thickened, thus leading to visual loss. Severe pain not helped by analgesia, ocular tenderness, diplopia and painful eye movements, due to a combination of extraocular muscle insertion on inflamed sclera and inflammation of the muscles (myositis).
- *Examination:* dilated fundoscopy to exclude exudative retinal detachments, uveal effusions, choroidal folds and disc oedema; B-scan ocular ultrasonography to show thickened posterior sclera and the 'T-sign' from fluid in Tenon's space.
- *Investigations:* the underlying cause is non-infective and immune related. Investigate Rh factor, ANA, p-ANCA and c-ANCA.
- *Management:* nonsteroidal anti-inflammatory drugs (NSAIDs) (for non-necrotising disease) and corticosteroids, delivered topically, periocularly, orally or intravenously (all if necrotising disease is present). Liaise with the rheumatologists to diagnose and treat an underlying systemic condition and advise if long-term steroid-sparing agents are indicated.

Advanced keratitis

An opaque cornea with severe reduction in visual acuity. Many causes and predisposing factors:

- Contact lens (CL) wear in bacterial keratitis and acanthamoebal keratitis.
- Previous herpes simplex and herpes zoster viral infections in viral keratitis.
- Patient who are from a hot, tropical country or who have experienced recent trauma in fungal keratitis.
- Loss of corneal sensation in neurotrophic keratitis. Always assess corneal sensation **prior** to instilling topical anaesthesia.
- The inability to close the eye (lagophthalmus) in exposure keratitis.

Treatment depends on the underlying aetiology and the patient requires regular vision monitoring in the first week following diagnosis.

Peripheral ulcerative keratitis (PUK)

This is associated with immune complex deposition in the peripheral cornea and subsequent damage to the stroma via the release of matrix metalloproteinases. Commonly due to rheumatoid arthritis and Wegener's granulomatosis. If the cause cannot be identified, the idiopathic version is called Mooren's ulcer. Patients will require systemic immunomodulators and may require keratoplasty.

Figure 19.1 Anterior ischaemia optic neuropathy (see Chapter 56)

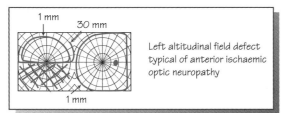

Left altitudinal field defect typical of anterior ischaemic optic neuropathy

Table 19.1 Aetiology of optic neuritis

Typical	Idiopathic Multiple sclerosis is the most common cause of retrobulbar neuritis
Atypical	Infectious (viral) Post infectious Granulomatous Autoimmune Contiguous inflammation of orbit, sinuses or meninges

Figure 19.2 In optic neuritis or retrobulbar neuritis, patients may have (a) reduced clour vision and/or (b) swollen optic disc

(a)

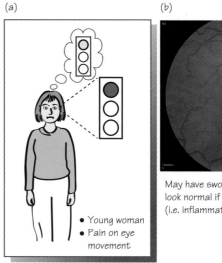

- Young woman
- Pain on eye movement

(b)

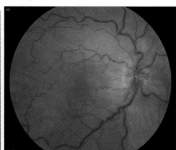

May have swollen optic nerve or look normal if retrobulbar neuritis (i.e. inflammation behind globe)

Figure 19.3 Migraine

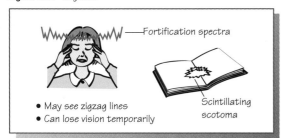

Fortification spectra

Scintillating scotoma

- May see zigzag lines
- Can lose vision temporarily

Figure 19.4 Idiopathic intracranial hypertension (IIH)

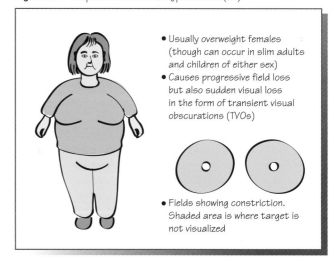

- Usually overweight females (though can occur in slim adults and children of either sex)
- Causes progressive field loss but also sudden visual loss in the form of transient visual obscurations (TVOs)

- Fields showing constriction. Shaded area is where target is not visualized

Figure 19.5 Haemorrhage from pituitary tumour

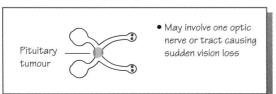

Pituitary tumour

- May involve one optic nerve or tract causing sudden vision loss

Ophthalmology at a Glance, Second Edition. Jane Olver, Lorraine Cassidy, Gurjeet Jutley, and Laura Crawley. © 2014 Jane Olver, Lorraine Cassidy, Gurjeet Jutley and Laura Crawley. Published 2014 by John Wiley & Sons, Ltd. Companion Website: www.ataglanceseries.com/ophthal

An adult patient presenting with sudden loss of vision but no inflammation (i.e. has a normal-looking white eye) should be suspected of having giant cell arteritis (GCA) (see Chapter 56); however, you should also exclude other causes, which are discussed in this chapter.

Aims

• Identify the main causes of sudden painful loss of vision in a white eye.

• Note that the pain may be ocular, cranial or both.

Sudden loss of vision associated with eye pain or headache in the white non-inflamed eye needs urgent attention as it may be due to life-threatening illness. The frequency of each disease varies between age groups.

Giant cell arteritis or temporal arteritis

Consider this as a diagnosis if there is visual disturbance with headache in patients over the age of 50. See Chapter 56 on GCA, and look at the visual field defect seen in anterior ischaemic optic neuropathy (AION) (Figure 19.1).

See also Chapter 53, 'Optic Nerve Disease', which shows the different types of visual field defects in papilloedema and pituitary tumour, and Chapter 55, 'Visual Field Defects', which shows the whole array of visual field defects in optic nerve and neurological disease.

Optic neuritis or retrobulbar neuritis

(Figure 19.2 and Table 19.1)

This is visual disturbance with eye pain, commonly in young adult people (particularly women). There are two clinical entities:

• Papillitis
  ◦ Inflammation of the actual optic nerve head.
  ◦ It appears swollen if all the nerve is affected (Figure 19.2b).
• Retrobulbar neuritis
  ◦ The part of the nerve behind the globe (i.e. the retrobulbar part of the nerve) is affected.
  ◦ There is sparing of the nerve head (see Figure 11.4 for an image of a normal optic disc).
  ◦ The patient will have the same symptoms and signs of optic nerve dysfunction, including reduced visual acuity, red desaturation and a relative afferent papillary defect. However, the disc appears normal in the acute phase.

Optic neuritis (ON) is closely linked with multiple sclerosis (MS), an inflammatory disease of the myelin sheaths in neurons of the central nervous system. Up to 50% of patients with MS will develop an episode of ON. Up to 30% of patients presenting with a first episode of ON will have underlying MS.

Typically, patients with ON present with:

• Sudden loss of vision
  ◦ Ranges from complete loss of vision to alteration in colour perception (e.g. the patient may complain of colours looking 'washed out' with the affected eye; Figure 19.2a).
• Eye pain
  ◦ Induced by eye movement.
• Other symptoms are attributable to undiagnosed demyelination, such as:
  ◦ paraesthesia
  ◦ bladder or bowel dysfunction
  ◦ limb weakness.

The course and treatment of ON came from the Optic Neuritis Treatment Trial in the 1990s. This was a randomized controlled trial consisting of three arms:

1 Intravenous corticosteroids.
2 Oral corticosteroids.
3 Placebo.

The following information was ascertained:

• There was a 28% probability of recurrence of ON in either eye in 5 years.

• Magnetic resonance imaging (MRI) of the brain is the single most important determinant of risk of developing MS by showing demyelinating plaques.

• Oral steroids are not required in isolated ON.

• Intravenous corticosteroids do have a place in clinical management, but their use is patient dependent. They may accelerate visual recovery but won't improve visual outcome in the long term. Particularly consider if:
  ◦ Vision is compromised in both eyes.
  ◦ There is severe pain.

• After an episode of ON, full return of visual function is never complete. Visual recovery begins rapidly within 2 weeks in most ON without treatment, but it continues to improve for up to 1 year.

Migraine

This is visual disturbance with headache.

These visual disturbances most commonly present as fortification spectra or scintillating scotoma, but occasionally as field loss or even total loss of vision, which recovers (Figure 19.3). There is often a family history of migraine.

Idiopathic intracranial hypertension (IIH)

Patients with IIH present with headache and transient visual obscurations (TVOs) (Figure 19.4). TVOs last for a few seconds, are unilateral or bilateral and are usually precipitated by movement or postural changes. They are pathognomonic of papilloedema.

• IIH occurs typically in obese females, but it can affect slim individuals of either sex as well as children.

• The optic discs are both swollen, and there is field loss.

• An MRI should be performed to exclude a space-occupying lesion and magnetic resonance angiography to exclude venous sinus thrombosis or an arteriovenous malformation affecting the venous sinuses.

• Thyroid dysfunction is a cause and must be excluded.

• Patients should be referred for urgent treatment, as this disease often results in permanent loss of the visual field.

• Treatment includes:
  ◦ Conservative: weight loss; stop any medications that may cause IIH (e.g. NSAIDs or tetracyclines).
  ◦ Medical: acetazolamide.
  ◦ Surgical: lumbo- or ventriculo-peritoneal shunt, or optic nerve sheath fenestration.

Haemorrhage associated with pituitary tumour

Rarely, a small haemorrhage in an undiagnosed pituitary tumour can cause sudden loss of vision associated with headache (Figure 19.5). Such patients require *urgent* referral to a neurosurgical unit, as this is a precursor of pituitary apoplexy.

KEY POINTS

• Painful loss of vision in a quiet eye may have a systemic cause (e.g. GCA).

• Retrobulbar neuritis—the disc looks normal in the acute phase.

• Idiopathic intracranial hypertension—both discs are swollen.

Figure 20.1 Vitreous haemorrhage

- i.e. from neovascularization in diabetes
- Vitreous haemorrhage

Figure 20.2 Age-related macular degeneration. (a) Disciform scar and (b) a sudden haemorrhage may cause sudden loss of vision

(a)
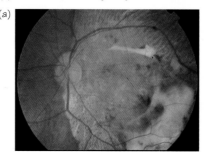

(b)
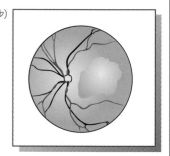

Figure 20.3 Retinal detachment

(a)
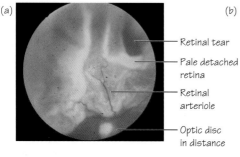

- Retinal tear
- Pale detached retina
- Retinal arteriole
- Optic disc in distance

(b)
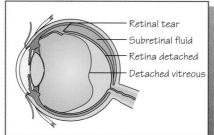

- Retinal tear
- Subretinal fluid
- Retina detached
- Detached vitreous

Symptoms
- Sudden visual loss preceded by floaters and flashes (photopsia)

Figure 20.4 (a) and (b) Central retinal vein occlusion

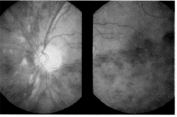

NB Check
- Intraocular pressure
- BP
- Viscosity

(a) Central or branch retinal vein occlusion – this is a sub-total CRVO or 3 quadrant BRVO

(b)
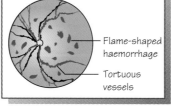

- Flame-shaped haemorrhage
- Tortuous vessels

Figure 20.5 (a) and (b) Central retinal artery occlusion

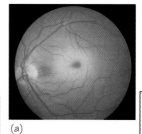

NB Check
- BP
- Pulse ?Afibrillation
- Carotids ?Bruit
- Heart ?Murmur
Refer to cardiologist

(a)

(b)
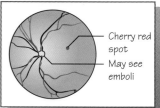

- Cherry red spot
- May see emboli

Figure 20.6 Vascular anatomy. (a) Anterior optic nerve supply and (b) vascular cast

(a)
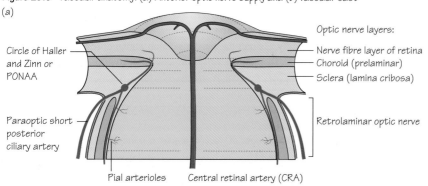

- Circle of Haller and Zinn or PONAA
- Paraoptic short posterior ciliary artery
- Pial arterioles
- Central retinal artery (CRA)

Optic nerve layers:
- Nerve fibre layer of retina
- Choroid (prelaminar)
- Sclera (lamina cribosa)
- Retrolaminar optic nerve

(b)
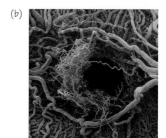

Vascular cast: Circle of Haller and Zinn or perioptic nerve arteriolar anastomosis (PONAA) *Copyright J Olver*

Ophthalmology at a Glance, Second Edition. Jane Olver, Lorraine Cassidy, Gurjeet Jutley, and Laura Crawley. © 2014 Jane Olver, Lorraine Cassidy, Gurjeet Jutley and Laura Crawley. Published 2014 by John Wiley & Sons, Ltd. Companion Website: www.ataglanceseries.com/ophthal

52

This is an alarming event. You can usually diagnose the cause by looking at the retina with an ophthalmoscope, or by doing visual fields.

Aim

Identify the main causes of painless loss of vision, in particular:
- Vitreous or sub-retinal haemorrhage
- Retinal detachment
- Types of vascular occlusion.

Vitreous and sub-retinal haemorrhage

(Figure 20.1)

Haemorrhage into the vitreous cavity can result in sudden painless loss of vision. The extent of visual loss will depend on the degree of haemorrhage.
- A large vitreous haemorrhage will cause total visual loss and loss of the red reflex or severe dulling of it, without a clear retinal view.
- A small vitreous haemorrhage will present as floaters and normal or only slightly reduced visual acuity.
- A sub-retinal haemorrhage has a distinct shape and is seen as a central dark scotoma using the Amsler chart.

Aetiology

- Proliferative retinopathy
  - Spontaneous rupture of abnormal fragile new vessels that grow on the retinal surface cause bleeding into the vitreous cavity.
  - Any ischaemia can cause neovascularization, including vein occlusions.
- Retinal detachment
  - A small retinal blood vessel may rupture when the retinal break occurs, bleeding into the vitreous cavity.
- Trauma
- Posterior vitreous detachment
  - Can result in vitreous haemorrhage if, as the vitreous separates from the retina, it pulls and ruptures a small blood vessel.
- Age-related macular degeneration (AMD) (Figure 20.2)—a haemorrhage may occur into the vitreous from the abnormally weak vessels forming a sub-retinal neovascular membrane (see Chapter 44). More often, it causes a sub-retinal haemorrhage.

Management

Referral to an ophthalmologist to determine cause and manage any complications (e.g. glaucoma due to red blood cells clogging up trabecular meshwork) that may occur. Treatment may be possible with laser or intravitreous injection.

Retinal detachment (Figure 20.3 and see Chapter 42)

- There are three distinctive types associated with different diseases:
  - Rhegmatogenous: secondary to a retinal tear.
  - Exudative: secondary to inflammation or vascular abnormalities.
  - Tractional: secondary to fibrovascular tissue caused by inflammation or neovascularization (such as proliferative diabetic retinopathy).
- All of these lead to sudden (sometimes gradual) painless loss of vision.
- Usually preceded by symptoms of flashing lights (photopsia) and/or floaters and/or visual field defects.
- When the macula is not involved (macula-on), the visual loss involves the peripheral field and visual acuity may be normal. Macula-

on detachment is regarded as an emergency as surgery done before the macula detaches can result in retention of good vision.

Once the macula is involved (macula-off), the central vision is lost.

A macular hole can result from a vitreous detachment and have only a very small amount of sub-retinal fluid around it.

- **Always** take a new flurry of floaters and/or photopsia **very** seriously. These patients need indentation with indirect ophthalmoscopy to exclude peripheral retinal breaks.
- When examining these patients with retinal detachment, include looking at the anterior third of the vitreous with the slit lamp. Look for pigmented cells floating around, the so-called tobacco dust or Shaffer's sign. By definition, if one can see the retinal pigmented cells in the vitreous, there must have been a retinal break. **So**, if you see tobacco dust and are unable to identify a break in the retina, you must get a senior ophthalmologist to review and locate the break.

Peripheral retinal tear

Management consists of laser to retinal hole (retinopexy) ± vitrectomy (within 24h if macula-on). Prior to surgery, it is important to ensure the patient's posture: if the detachment is temporal, ensure that the patient lies with the contralateral cheek to the pillow. If the detachment is in the nasal retina, ensure that the patient lies with the ipsilateral cheek to the pillow.

Macula hole

Vitrectomy and epiretinal peel, if indicated.

Vascular occlusion (see Chapters 47 and 48)

Patients with retinal vascular occlusions often present with sudden painless loss of vision.

Central retinal vein occlusion (CRVO; Figure 20.4) or branch retinal vein occlusion (BRVO)

Aetiology
- Systemic hypertension
- Raised intraocular pressure
- Hyperviscosity syndromes
- Vessel wall disease (e.g. diabetes, or inflammation such as sarcoidosis).

> **WARNING**
> ▶ Check blood pressure, examine for arteriosclerosis, check intraocular pressure and exclude diabetes and systemic inflammation.
> ▶ In young patients presenting with CRVO or BRVO, or older patients where there is no obvious cause, exclude hyperviscosity syndromes.

Central retinal artery occlusion (CRAO; Figure 20.5) or a branch retinal artery occlusion

Aetiology
- Very high intraocular pressure, usually great than 30 mmHg
- Arterial embolus from diseased carotid, valvular heart disease or atrial fibrillation
- Arterial occlusion from atheroma or inflammation (e.g. giant cell arteritis).

> **WARNING**
> ▶ All patients with CRAO need a full cardiovascular work-up.

Non-arteritic anterior or posterior ischaemic optic neuropathy (AION or PION, respectively)

(see also Chapter 19)

• Results from occlusion or hypoperfusion of the small blood vessels supplying the optic nerve head (AION) or posterior optic nerve (PION). See the diagram vessels and ocular cast of the circle of Haller and Zinn (Figure 20.6).

• In AION, the optic disc is swollen; this swelling may be segmental or involve the entire nerve head. There are usually associated splinter haemorrhages at the disc.

• In PION, the optic disc looks normal.

• There may be arteriosclerosis and arteriovenous nipping, depending on the cause.

• Risk factors: arteriosclerosis, hypertension, a hypotensive episode, smoking and a 'disc at risk' (e.g. a small optic nerve head with no central cup).

Cerebral

Cerebrovascular accident (CVA)

A haemorrhagic or thrombo-embolic CVA affecting the visual pathways will present as acute painless visual loss. Depending on the site of the lesion, the patient will have a corresponding field defect on fields to confrontation.

Acephalgic migraine

This rare form of migraine presents with transient visual disturbances involving one or both eyes in the absence of headaches.

KEY POINTS

• Retinal detachment is an ocular cause of sudden painless loss of vision.

• Central retinal vein occlusion is commonly caused by systemic hypertension.

• Central retinal artery occlusion may be caused by giant cell arteritis.

---

21 Gradual loss of vision

Figure 21.1 Uncorrected refractive error

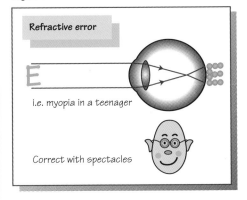

Refractive error

i.e. myopia in a teenager

Correct with spectacles

Figure 21.2 (a) and (b) Cataract

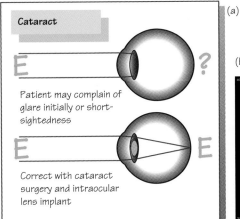

Cataract

Patient may complain of glare initially or short-sightedness

Correct with cataract surgery and intraocular lens implant

(a)

(b)

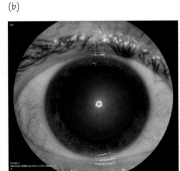

Figure 21.3 Glaucoma. (a) Diagrammatic and (b) optic disc cupping

(a)

Primary open angle glaucoma

Causes progressive visual field loss
Intraocular pressure (IOP) elevated
+ 21 mmHg

30 mmHg

Cupped disc

Treat with ocular antihypertensives

(b)

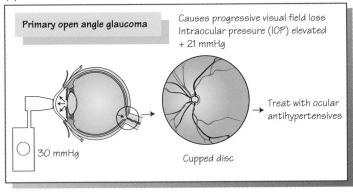

Figure 21.4 Diabetic retinopathy. (a) Treatment with a laser and (b) diabetic maculopathy – the white circles are laser burns

(a)

(b)

Retinal disease

Treat with laser

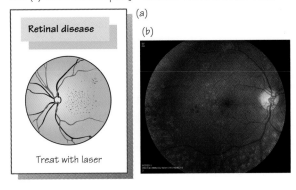

Figure 21.5 Colour fundus photograph of right eye showing a large area of geographical atrophy at the macula

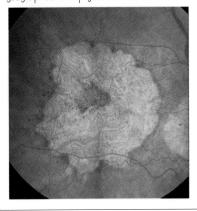

TIP

Elderly patients with cataract may also have ageing macular degeneration and the contribution of each to their gradual painless loss of vision must be established prior to offering cataract surgery, or they may not get an optimum result

Ophthalmology at a Glance, Second Edition. Jane Olver, Lorraine Cassidy, Gurjeet Jutley, and Laura Crawley. © 2014 Jane Olver, Lorraine Cassidy, Gurjeet Jutley and Laura Crawley. Published 2014 by John Wiley & Sons, Ltd. Companion Website: www.ataglanceseries.com/ophthal

Be suspicious of the presence of these common conditions:
- uncorrected refractive error
- cataract
- chronic simple glaucoma
- retinal disease
- tumour.

Aim
- Identify the common causes of gradual painless loss of vision in a white eye.
- Particularly consider the age of the patient when trying to figure out the cause.

When a patient presents with a gradual painless loss of vision, the cause will often vary with age, as certain conditions can be more common in certain age groups (e.g. cataract and ageing maculopathy in the elderly).

Refractive error (Figure 21.1; see also Chapters 8, 9 and 35)
- Undetected and uncorrected refractive error is a common cause of gradual visual loss in all age groups.
- Emmetropia means one can achieve 6/6 visual acuity unaided. In this situation, light rays are refracted (bent) by both the cornea and lens, and are **in focus on the retina**. Note that the cornea has two-thirds of the total refractive power of the eye.
- In myopia, light rays are refracted to a **focal point anterior to the retina** (somewhere in the vitreous) and so are blurred. Causes are:
  - Axial: when the eye is abnormally long.
  - Refractive: whereby the power of refraction is increased either due to the:
    - Cornea, such as in the condition keratoconus; or
    - Lens, particularly when nuclear sclerotic cataracts cause a so-called 'myopic shift'.
- Traditionally, concave spectacles and/or contact lenses correct myopia. More recently, with higher patient expectations, refractive surgery has become more en vogue. In the United Kingdom, the most common procedure is LASIK (laser-assisted in situ keratomileusis), whereby a partial thickness (lamellar) circular flap and hinge are created by a femto-laser. An excimer laser is used to reshape the bared stroma and the flap replaced. See Chapter 35.
- In hypermetropia, the light rays are refracted to a **focal point behind the retina**. Again, the causes can be split into:
  - Axial: whereby the eye is short in length. This explains why children with their small developing eyes are hypermetropic.
  - Refractive: seen sometimes after complicated cataract surgery, if the patient is left without a lens (aphakic).
- As healthcare professionals, the most common refractive errors we encounter are:
  - Hypermetropia in young children.
  - Axial myopia in teenagers and young adults.
  - Refractive myopia in older patients.

The young children group is the most important as they often don't complain at all and amblyopia may have occurred prior to presentation (see Chapter 23).

Astigmatism
- The cornea is usually spherical in shape, and hence rays of light from all directions are refracted equally onto one focal point. In an astigmatic cornea, the cornea is more rugby ball shaped, whereby one axis is steep and the axis at 90° to this is gentle. Hence, the ability to bend light rays differs in different meridians of the cornea, and rather than one focal point being achieved, there are many, leading to a blurred image. The multiple focal points comprise Sturm's conoid. Physiologically in younger patients, there is an element of astigmatism due to the eye being 'squashed' between the orbital floor and the brow. Astigmatism is treated with a toric lens, which is a spherical lens, with a superimposed cylindrical lens to steepen the gentler axis.

Presbyopia
- The amazing ability of the human eye is only too evident in considering how one is able to focus objects both near and from a distance. This characteristic of the lens to adopt a more fattened shape (upon relaxation of the zonules) to bring near objects into focus is called accommodation. In youth, the lens can accommodate up to 15–20 dioptres. Beyond 45 years, this ability diminishes to 1 dioptre, clinically termed presbyopia. We treat this condition with spectacle correction for both near and distance, either separately or with one pair of glasses (bifocals or verifocals).

Cataract (Figure 21.2; see also Chapters 36, 37 and 38)
Vision depends on clear windows so that light can reach the retina: thus, opacities in cornea, lens and vitreous will impair VA. Most commonly, the opacity occurs in the lens (i.e. cataract).
- Cataract commonly causes gradual loss of vision in the elderly. They may notice nothing at all and the presence of an early cataract is detected by their optician, or they will have a gradual blurring of distant, then near, vision. If the cataract is placed posterior in the lens as a plaque (posterior sub-capsular lens opacity), they will notice glare and reduced vision in bright sunlight, with improved vision indoors.
- It may also occur in younger age groups who are at risk (e.g. patients with diabetes, on steroids, with chronic uveitis and/or with a family history of cataract).
- Cataract may also occur in young children (congenital cataract). It is very important to check the red reflex of any child who presents with reduced vision, and any baby who does not fix and follow, as they require urgent treatment with patching and glasses to prevent amblyopia (see Chapter 23). Some congenital cataracts do not significantly interfere with vision (e.g. blue dot cataract).

Modern cataract surgery is performed through small incisions at the surgical limbus. The technique of choice is phacoemulsification and implanting a foldable intraocular lens. Throughout specialist training in the United Kingdom, we are exposed to increasingly difficult cataracts and are expected to have performed 350 operations at completion of training.

Glaucoma (Figure 21.3; see also Chapters 39, 40 and 41)
Primary open-angle glaucoma (POAG)
- Causes slowly progressive glaucomatous optic neuropathy and painless visual field loss.

- Risk factors include Afro-Caribbean origin and family history of POAG.
- Patients are usually completely unaware that they have open-angle glaucoma, and it is detected by their optician finding raised intraocular pressure or noticing a cupped disc.
- By the time a patient with glaucoma presents with visual symptoms, 90% of the nerve fibre layer is destroyed.
- Glaucoma screening will often pick up POAG before any severe damage has occurred, and many patients are maintained on topical medication without significant progression or the need for drainage surgery (see Chapter 40).

Retinal disease (see Chapters 44 and 45)

This should be considered in the patient with none of the above causes of reduced vision. It occurs particularly in patients at risk:
- Diabetics (diabetic retinopathy; Figure 21.4)
- Hypertensives (hypertensive retinopathy)
- The elderly (age-related macular degeneration (AMD)). This is the commonest cause of blindness in the elderly, in which their central vision for reading, colour and fine detail is affected (Figure 21.5).
- Children or young adults with neurometabolic diseases or a family history of retinal disease (e.g. retinitis pigmentosa).
- Previous history of an intraocular foreign body (IOFB) may cause the development of siderosis bulbi; this is a condition where iron from an IOFB that has not been removed can cause retinal toxicity. The patient presents years after the initial injury with gradual loss of vision. The iris in the affected eye of a blue-eyed individual may have a greenish hue.

- Individuals taking medications known to cause drug-induced macular disease (e.g. chloroquine, hydroxychloroquine, tamoxifen, chlorpromazine, thioridazine or vigabatrin).

Tumours (see also Chapter 19, 31 and 55)

Any tumour that affects the visual pathway may cause symptoms of gradual, painless loss of vision by pressure on the optic nerve or eye. Examples include:
- Intraocular tumour (e.g. choroidal malignant melanoma or choroidal metastases from the breast or prostate in adults, or retinoblastoma in children)
- Intraocular lymphoma, which may masquerade as bilateral intermediate uveitis
- Tumour of the optic nerve (e.g. meningioma or glioma)
- Tumour of the orbit or optic nerve (e.g. orbital lymphoma, sphenoidal wing meningioma or dysthyroid eye disease)
- Any brain tumour involving the visual pathways (e.g. pituitary tumour or occipital lobe tumour).

These are not common and should always be considered when no other cause can be found.

KEY POINTS

- Myopia is common in young teenagers.
- Patients with POAG are usually unaware of their disease.
- Cataract and ageing maculopathy cause decreased vision in the elderly.
- Tumours are a rare cause of gradual visual loss.

Figure 22.1 Testing visual acuity in newborns up to 2 months old

(a) Fix and follow. In the newborn see if they will fix and follow a shiny colourful target

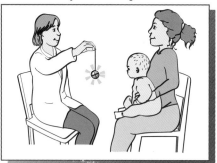

(b) Spinning. Another way of getting a crude idea of vision is to pick the child up, and hold him at arm's length and spin him around in a circle

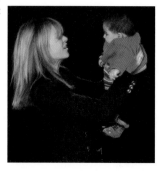

(c) More advanced ways of checking a newborn's vision include forced choice preferential looking, a clinical test

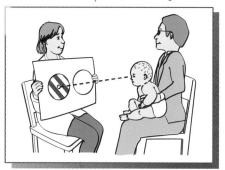

(d) Electrophysiological testing with visual evoked potentials (VEPs) /visual evoked responses (VERs)

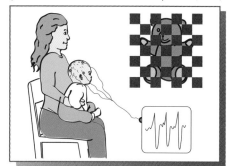

Figure 22.2 Testing visual acuity in infants and toddler up to 3 years old

(a)

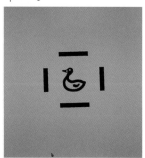

In the pre-verbal infant, vision can be assessed as for the newborn. Older infants can see picture optotyes of familiar objects (fish, apple, boat)

(b)

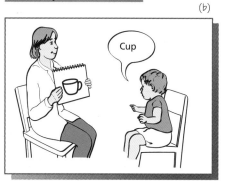

Cup

Figure 22.3 Testing visual acuity in 4–5 year olds. Children should wear this type of glasss to ensure that monocular vision is tested

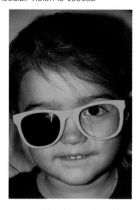

Depending on social background and learning ability most 4 and 5 year olds will be able to match letters, and some children at this age can even read letters. For children who cannot read letters the "Sheridan–Gardner singles" test is used

Ophthalmology at a Glance, Second Edition. Jane Olver, Lorraine Cassidy, Gurjeet Jutley, and Laura Crawley. © 2014 Jane Olver, Lorraine Cassidy, Gurjeet Jutley and Laura Crawley. Published 2014 by John Wiley & Sons, Ltd. Companion Website: www.ataglanceseries.com/ophthal

Before children can speak they can see, and surprisingly, we can measure their visual acuity fairly accurately using the tests described in this chapter.

Aim

How to assess visual acuity in different aged children.

Visual development

A child's vision continues to develop after birth and maturation. Normal visual development in both eyes is important for children to perceive the world, their education and their social interactions. An infant who appears not to see well may have **delayed visual maturation** or a more serious cause. Measuring visual acuity in children requires skill and patience, but even simple techniques can be used to elicit vision and reassure the parent.

It is important to detect amblyopia, as this can be treated by glasses and/or patching if discovered early enough. See Chapter 23.

Newborn child up to 2 months (Figure 22.1)

Assessment of vision in the neonate is dependent on the age and behavioural state of the child. When a child is pre-verbal, you depend on his/her eye movements for information about visual function. At 6 weeks of age, children are able to smile. Without making any noise, smile at the child, and if the child smiles back, you know they can see!

A number of techniques are used to test vision in newborns:

Fix and follow

• Use a pen torch or large brightly coloured silent toy to see if the child fixes and follows.
• With the child sitting on the mother's knee, move the toy *slowly* from left to right about 33 cm in front of the child's face. If the child can see, they will follow the toy only if awake and if the toy is moved slowly as eye movements are immature at this age.
• If possible, test each eye separately by occluding one eye with an occlusive patch.
• If the child fixes and follows the target, record the vision as '**fixes and follows**'.
• If the child doesn't follow the toy, this may be because they can't see, is drowsy or is just not interested; therefore, try again later.

Spinning baby test

Whilst **spinning** the child, observe his eye movements. The spinning will cause a conjugate deviation (nystagmus) in the opposite direction to the rotation if he can see. This is the vestibulo-ocular reflex (VOR). When you stop spinning, there is a post-rotational nystagmus. If the nystagmus persists after a few seconds, the child may be severely visually impaired or have a cortical lesion.

Other clinical tests

Preferential looking

• Cards have different-sized grating patterns on the right or left half of the card and are plain on the other half of each card. The card is shown to the infant, who will look towards the grating side if she can see it.

Visual evoked potentials (VEPs)

• The child has electrodes on her head which record brain signals if she sees the pattern on the screen.

Infants up to 3 years of age (Figure 22.2)
Cardiff Acuity Test

• Another way of recording vision in these infants is to use the Cardiff Acuity Test, frequently referred to as Cardiff Cards (CCs) in clinical practice (Figure 22.2a).
• Each card has a line drawing of a familiar object on either the upper or lower half of the card, and the thickness of the lines varies. According to the thickness of the line, the card will have a letter (e.g. CC H) with a Snellen and LogMAR equivalent on the back for the examiner to see (e.g. 6/6 Snellen or 0.00 LogMAR for the finest line).
• From a distance of 50 cm or 1 m, the cards are rapidly shown to the child and the examiner observes the child making vertical eye movements up and down to the location of the picture. For example, visual acuity is recorded as 'CC H at 50 cm–Snellen Equivalent 6/9'. If possible, the acuity of each eye should be recorded separately.

Toddler (18 months–4 years)

Once the child can speak, you can use a subjective vision test and ask him to verbally identify some simple and familiar pictures.

Single and Crowded LogMAR Kay Picture Tests

• The most common method of assessing vision in this group is with the Kay Picture Test (Figure 22.2b).
• The Single LogMAR Kay Picture Test consists of a spiral-bound book of cards. On each page, there is a single black line drawing of a picture on a white background which can usually be recognized by children from 18 months old.
• The Crowded LogMAR Kay Picture Test consists of a larger spiral-bound book of cards, on each of which there are four line picture drawings in a rectangular box on a white background. This allows for a linear visual acuity with a crowding effect for increased testing sensitivity, which can be used prior to the child learning letters. This test is recommended from 3 years old.
• For both the Single and Crowded Kay Picture Test books, each line drawing has a Snellen and LogMAR equivalent depending on the size of the drawing (i.e. the largest drawing is equivalent to the 6/60 letter on the Snellen chart).
• The examiner stands 3 m from the child and asks her to identify each picture.
• The child can name the pictures, or if she is unable or too shy to name them, she can match the pictures using a matching card held by the child or by the parent that she is sitting with.

Young children (4–5 years)
Keeler Crowded LogMAR Test

• The Keeler Crowded LogMAR Test consists of a box containing two crowded books and one uncrowded book.
• In the crowded books, each page has four letters of one size.
• The examiner stands 3 m away and presents letters on the card.
• The child is asked to name the letters. If the child is unable to name the letters, he is given a matching card to use instead.
• Each eye is examined separately (Figure 22.3), and the acuity recorded.

KEY POINTS

• In newborn children, use 'fix and follow' or the spinning baby test to elicit the presence of vision.
• In infants younger than 2 years old, use the Cardiff Cards.
• In infants aged 2–3 years, use a Kay Picture Test.
• In children aged 4–5 years, use the Keeler Crowded LogMAR Test.

23 Strabismus (squints)

Examination

Figure 23.1 Corneal Hirschberg reflection test

To detect a strabismus the **corneal reflex** position is observed – each mm of displacement is equal to about 15 prism dioptres (7 degrees)

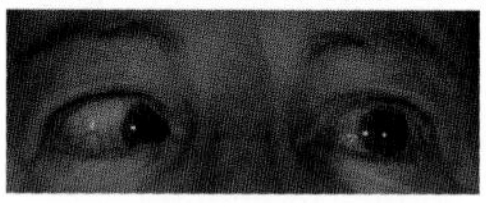

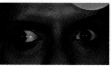

Example: Right 45 prism dioptre convergent strabismus (esotropia)

Figure 23.3 Right exotropia (divergent strabismus)

When the left fixing eye is covered with an opaque occluder, the right eye moves inwards to take up fixation of the target. The strabismus is divergent (exotropia)

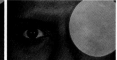

Figure 23.4 Prism bar measurement
The size of the strabismus is measured with a prism bar

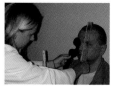

Prism alternate cover test

Figure 23.5 Eye movements. Assessment of nine positions of gaze (primary and eight directions)

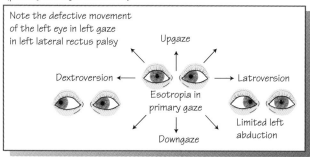

Note the defective movement of the left eye in left gaze in left lateral rectus palsy

Upgaze
Dextroversion
Latroversion
Esotropia in primary gaze
Limited left abduction
Downgaze

Figure 23.2 The cover tests

(a) The cover–uncover test – to detect the presence of a strabismus:
- Observe if one eye is preferred for fixation
- Ask the patient to look at the fixation target – if in a child this can be a light or toy
- Occlude (for a few seconds) the eye that appears to be fixing. As you cover the eye, watch the other uncovered eye to see if it moves to take up fixation
- Remove the occluder and see if the original eye retakes up fixation. If it does, it is the preferred fixating eye and the other eye has a strabismus (non-alternating heterotropia)
- Do this for near and then distance vision

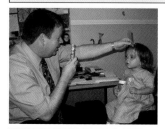

(b) The alternate cover test – to detect a latent strabismus or phoria in a patient with straight eyes on cover test:
- Ask the patient to fixate on an object
- Cover one eye then rapidly move cover to the other eye
- Repeat rapidly several times
- Observe the movement of the covered eye as it becomes uncovered
- If it moves inwards to take up fixation the patient has an 'exophoria'
- Do test for near and then distance
Also can be used with a prism bar to measure the maximum size of a strabismus

KEY POINTS

- Esotropia is a convergent strabismus
- Amblyopia must be treated early – ideally before the age of 5 years
- Beware: strabismus may be a presentaion of an intracranial tumour or retinoblastoma

Treatment

Figure 23.6 Glasses. (a) Convergent strabismus (esotropia) – left accommodative esotropia and (b) long-sight (hypermetropia) fully corrected by wearing hypermetropic glasses

(a)
(b)

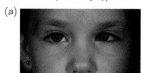

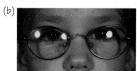

Figure 23.7 Patching. The left good eye is patched in order to encourage use of the right amblyopic eye

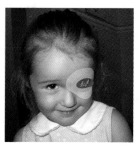

You will find that the terms 'squint' and 'strabismus' are used interchangeably. Strabismus is the correct medical term. A child with strabismus can have a lazy (amblyopic) eye, whilst in an adult it can be indicative of a wide range of disorders: a cranial nerve palsy, tumour, trauma, thyroid eye disease or the like. In this chapter, we are concentrating on strabismus in children. Many of the principles of examination of a child also apply to an adult. For adult traumatic, restrictive and paralytic strabismus see Chapters 16, 29, 30 and 54, for more on adult strabismus, please see Chapter 28.

Aims

- Understand strabismus terminology.
- Do a cover test to detect strabismus.
- Know the basic principles of amblyopia therapy.

A child with strabismus will not 'grow out' of it. There may be a sinister cause such as cataract or retinoblastoma, so you should always do a red reflex and if there is a white reflex, this is indicative of more serious pathology. Any child suspected of having strabismus should be referred to an orthoptist for precise measurements and possible patching, and to an ophthalmologist for assessment, including refraction and for management.

Orthoptists are allied health professionals who assess patients with diplopia (double vision), strabismus and eye movement defects. They work closely with **ophthalmologists** in the management of children's visual development, testing paediatric visual acuity (see Chapter 22) and treating amblyopia.

Aetiology and pathophysiology

Concomitant strabismus

Concomitant means that the deviation remains the same in all positions of gaze.

- Binocular single vision (BSV) usually develops by 3–5 months old. If BSV does not 'lock in', esotropia (convergent strabismus) can develop at this time, although most concomitant strabismus develops later at around 2–4 years, particularly with hypermetropia (longsightedness requiring plus dioptre glasses).
- Any cause of reduced vision in one eye will interrupt BSV and result in strabismus, such as cataract, retinoblastoma or anisometropia (a difference of refraction between the two eyes).
- Children with a family history of strabismus or refractive error and those with developmental abnormalities have a higher incidence of concomitant squint.

Incomitant strabismus

Incomitant means that the angle of the deviated eye changes with position of the gaze and is not constant like in concomitant strabismus.

- Congenital causes are rare (e.g. third, fourth or sixth nerve palsy).

- Acquired incomitant strabismus presents with diplopia in adults. A child may adopt a compensatory head posture to minimize diplopia and therefore may not complain of diplopia. A very young child will suppress the second image and develop amblyopia if untreated.
- Acquired causes include cranial nerve palsy (paralytic) secondary to intracranial pathology, thyroid eye disease and post-traumatic orbital floor fracture (restrictive).

Management

Orthoptists, optometrists and ophthalmologists collaborate in the management of strabismus using a combination of glasses, surgery and orthoptic treatment.

Childhood concomitant and congenital incomitant strabismus

Role of the orthoptist:

- Measures visual acuity (VA).
- Detects and measures strabismus using the Hirschberg test (Figure 23.1), cover tests (Figures 23.2 and 23.3) and prism bar measurements (Figure 23.4).
- Assesses eye movements (Figure 23.5).
- Assesses binocular vision (including tests for stereopsis).
- Monitors amblyopia therapy with patching (Figure 23.7) ± atropine occlusion.

Refraction

The optometrist or ophthalmologist performs refraction (cycloplegic if child aged <7 years). In fully or partial accommodative esotropia with high hypermetropia (with dioptre glasses required), wearing glasses will fully or partially correct the deviation as well as improve visual acuity, and surgery may not be required (Figure 23.6).

Amblyopia therapy

Spectacles (if applicable) and a patch worn on the better eye for a specified number of hours per day, depending on the child's age and visual acuity (Figure 23.7). The patch completely covers the good eye to encourage the bad eye (amblyopic one) to be used and develop vision. This treatment method is generally unsuccessful after age 7 years.

Surgery

Strabismus surgery is performed if the strabismus is socially unacceptable and to restore or improve binocular vision. In esotropia, the horizontal rectus muscles are operated, recessing the medial rectus and resecting the lateral rectus or bimedial rectus recessions.

Acquired incomitant strabismus (children and adults)

- The underlying cause must be established and treated (e.g. intracranial tumour, diabetes or hypertension).
- Orthoptic management is by joining the diplopia with Fresnel prisms or prisms incorporated into the spectacle prescription (see Figure 9.3).
- Surgery is performed if BSV is not comfortably restored once the extraocular muscles recover or have been stable for at least 6 months.

Figure 24.1 Leukokoria
Leukokoria – a white coloured pupil – exclude congenital cataract or retinoblastoma

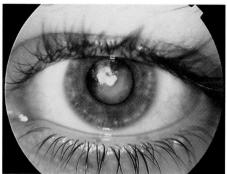

Figure 24.2 A coloboma is a hole in any structure of the eye and is due to the failure of the choroidal fissure to close during embryological development. It is associated with a mutation in the PAX2 gene. (a) Right eyelid coloboma and microphthalmos with partial cryptophthalmus (hidden eye), (b) a healthy red reflex through a dilated pupil with a small inferior coloboma and (c) a white retinal reflex and optic disc coloboma

(a)

(b)

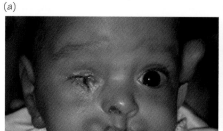

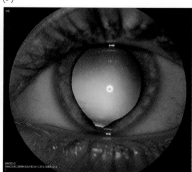

(c)

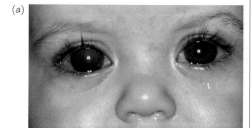

Figure 24.3 Retinopathy of prematurity (ROP). (a) Dragged disc, (b) proliferating retinal vessels on ridge and (c) there is an international classification of retinopathy of prematurity (ROP) where worsening stages are recognized. The retina is divided into zones for its development

(a)

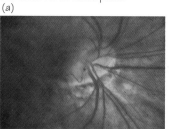

(b)

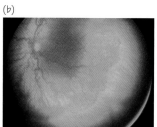

(c)

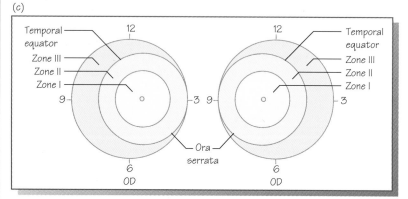

Figure 24.4 Congenital glaucoma (buphthalmos). (a) Buphthalmos: large, watering photophobic eyes with corneal clouding and (b) examination under anaesthesia and measurement of intraocular pressure using a handheld Perkins tonometer

(a)

(b)

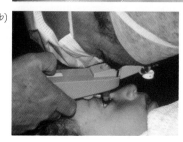

ROP zones

The area of retinal involvement in ROP can be divided anatomically into differing zones. One must make imaginary lines as follows:
- Zone 1 = Take the distance from the optic nerve to the fovea and multiply by two. This forms the radius of the circle for Zone 1
- Zone 2 = Take the distance from the optic nerve to the ora serrata (the peripheral edge of the retina), and use this as a radius for a circle. Zone 2 is this circle minus Zone 1
- Zone 3 = This is the residual temporal crescent, aside from Zone 2

Classification is based on:
- Anatomical involvement
- Staging (from a faint demarcation line all the way through to retinal detachment)
- The presence or absence of plus disease (vascular dilatation and tortuosity)

Ophthalmology at a Glance, Second Edition. Jane Olver, Lorraine Cassidy, Gurjeet Jutley, and Laura Crawley. © 2014 Jane Olver, Lorraine Cassidy, Gurjeet Jutley and Laura Crawley. Published 2014 by John Wiley & Sons, Ltd. Companion Website: www.ataglanceseries.com/ophthal

Aims

- Confidently check for a red reflex.
- Differential diagnosis of leukocoria.
- Main sight-threatening eye problems in neonates.

Leukocoria

Leukocoria is derived from the Greek words 'leuko' = white, and 'coria' = pupil, when noted an urgent referral is indicated.

Leukocoria is seen as a white-coloured pupillary reflex when an ophthalmoscope light is shone at the pupil (Figure 24.1). In a normal red reflex, the ophthalmoscope light bounces off the red-orange retina and an overall red reflex is seen. Leukocoria can indicate severe ocular pathology and be amblyogenic. Causes of leukocoria include the following.

Retinoblastoma (see also chapter 31)

- This malignant tumour of the retina is the most common intraocular tumour of childhood.
- It is the most sinister cause of leukocoria as it can potentially kill the child.
- Urgent assessment and treatment are required by a joint paediatric oncology and paediatric ophthalmology team in a specialist centre.
- Can be either hereditary (usually bilateral) or sporadic (usually unilateral).
- Treatment involves radioactive plaque or enucleation and adjuvant chemotherapy.
- 90–95% survival at 5 years with treatment.

Congenital cataract

- Presents as leukocoria, a dull red reflex, squint or nystagmus.
- If bilateral, the child may be visually inattentive.
- There is usually no relative afferent papillary defect unless there is other retinal or optic nerve pathology.
- Causes include idiopathic (most common), familial autosomal dominant, galactosaemia and rubella (also causes microcephaly, congenital heart defects, corneal clouding and retinopathy).
- Needs *urgent* (within days) assessment with a view to cataract surgery and subsequent amblyopia therapy. Some cataracts are small and need monitoring and amblyopia therapy.

Coloboma of the eye and eyelid (Figure 24.2)

Failure of the choroidal fissure to close during embryological development. It is associated with a mutation in the PAX2 gene.

A chorio-retinal coloboma or large optic disc coloboma (Figure 24.2c) can also give a white retinal reflex and is associated with severe amblyopia. Smaller colobomas of the iris (Figure 24.2b) can exist without affecting the posterior part of the eye and be associated with normal visual development.

Non-accidental injury (NAI)

- A neonate with leukocoria or any type of ocular trauma may have NAI.

Retinopathy of prematurity (ROP) (Figure 24.3)

- Pre term babies born at <30 weeks and with birth weight <1500 g are screened.
- Incomplete retinal vascularization leads to relative hypoxia causing new abnormal blood vessels to grow which leak and scar.
- Leukocoria is seen only in advanced disease due to a large tractional retinal detachment.
- The mainstay of treatment is ablation of the avascular retina and reduction of VEGF production with cryotherapy or laser.
- Recently, the Bevacizumab Eliminates the Angiogenic Threat of Retinopathy of Prematurity (Beat-ROP) study has shown that intravitreal bevacizumab has a role in treatment for zone 1 and stage 3 disease.
- Complications of treatment include cataract and myopia.
- In severe ROP with retinal detachment, vitreoretinal surgery is often only palliative.

Other less common causes of Leukorcoria

- familial exudative retinopathy
- Coat's disease
- infections: toxoplasmosis and toxocariasis
- hyperplastic primary persistent vitreous (HPPV).

Other neonatal ophthalmic conditions

- Ophthalmia neonatorum is a notifiable disease.
- The neonate usually has a unilateral or bilateral purulent conjunctivitis within a few days of birth.
- Take swabs for bacteria (including Gram and Giemsa stains), a *Chlamydia* immunofluorescent antibody test and viral culture.
- Suspect *Neisseria gonorrhoeae* (usually within 3 days of birth) or *Chlamydia trachomatis* (usually sub-acute from day 5 post-birth) until proved otherwise as both can cause blindness.
- Systemic and topical treatment is essential, as is the referral of both parents to a sexually transmitted disease (STD) clinic.

Buphthalmos

- A large eye in an infant associated with congenital glaucoma and a cause of blindness or defective vision (Figure 24.4a)
- The intraocular pressure can be measured with a handheld tono-pen or 'iCare' (Figure 24.4b).

Anophthalmos and microphthalmos

- Total absence of an eye (anophthalmos) or a very small ocular remnant (microphthalmos)
- The aim of management is to promote orbital bony development by keeping the ocular remnant (microphthalmos or cyst) and expanding the soft tissue of the orbit and eyelids sequentially. Eventually, an ocular prosthesis (artificial eye) can be made specific to the patient.

Watering eyes (epiphora) due to congenital nasolacrimal duct obstruction (NLDO) (also Chapter 25)

- Aetiology: opening of the lower end of the nasolacrimal duct (where it enters the nose in the inferior meatus at the valve of Hasner) is often delayed for several months.
- Note: an important differential for watery eyes in an infant is congenital glaucoma (assess for buphthalmos by measuring the diameter of the cornea).
- Treatment of congenital NLDO:
  ∘ Advise the parent that the watering is likely to resolve by age 1 year in 90% of cases.
  ∘ Apply daily small-finger massage over the lacrimal sac at the medial canthus to open the valve.
  ∘ An expressible mucocoele suggests nasolacrimal duct block requiring dacryocystorhinostomy surgery.
  ∘ For persistent watering over age 1 year, do a syringe and probing (S&P) under general anaesthesia. If recurrent repeat S&P and consider intubation or DCR.

Ptosis (also Chapter 25)

A neonate with an upper eyelid drooping across the visual axis is likely to have a weak levator palpebrae superioris (LPS) function. They should be referred urgently to an ophthalmologist with a view to urgent frontalis suspension surgery as this is an amblyogenic stimulus. Otherwise, wait until age 4 years if visual development is not threatened.

KEY POINTS

- Very important causes of leukocoriaare retinoblastoma, ROP and congenital cataract.
- A watering eye from congenital NLDO usually resolves age 1 year.
- Beware: congenital glaucoma may present in neonates with large or watery eyes.

Figure 25.1 Orbital, peri-orbital and eyelid haemangioma

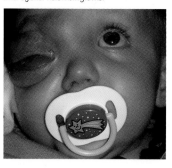

Figure 25.2 Inferior lid chalazion, also known as a meibomian cyst

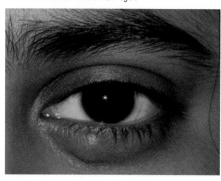

Figure 25.3 Molluscum contagiosum

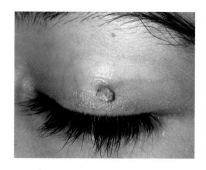

Figure 25.4 (a) Limbal dermoid

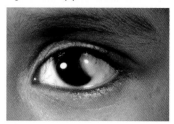

(b) Dermoid cyst

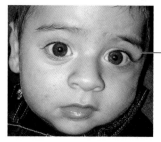

— Dermoid cyst

(c) Dermolipoma

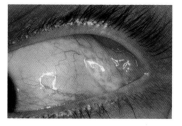

Figure 25.5 (a) Congenital left ptosis (b) and acquired ptosis, e.g from allergic vernal conjunctivitis, (c) everted upper eyelid showing giant papillae lumps

(a)

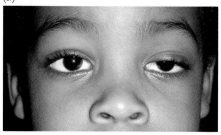

(b)

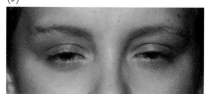

(c)

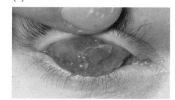

Severe orbital disease

Figure 25.6 Posterior orbital cellulitis. The patient's eyelid is closed and there are reduced eye movements. Urgent management is required.

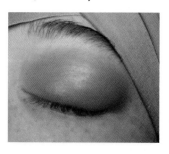

Figure 25.7 Rhabdomyosarcoma

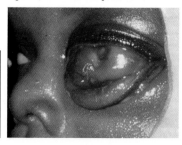

- Rare malignant orbital tumour of childhood that can metastasize. It may present as orbital cellulitis
- Average age of onset: 7 years
- Grows fast and progresses
- If suspected, urgent referral and biopsy required

Rhabdomyosarcoma (figure 25.7) and leukaemia are important differential diagnoses of bacterial orbital cellulitis

Aims

- Identify common paediatric eyelid, tear duct and orbital problems.
- Know why and when to operate on ptosis.
- Management of orbital cellulitis.

Eyelid lumps

Capillary haemangioma (Figure 25.1)

Swelling appears at birth or shortly afterwards, then increases in size for about 6 months. This is most common in the superonasal orbit and eyelid. It grows slowly, during which time it can cause mechanical ptosis and risk of amblyopia if the lid covers the visual axis or its weight causes astigmatism. This used to be treated with local infiltration of steroids to speed up resolution and reduce the bulk of the haemangioma, but it is now treated with oral beta-blockers. It usually spontaneously regresses after age 1 year.

Stye (external hordeolum)

- Lash follicle infection—hot red lump that resolves rapidly.

Chalazion (Figure 25.2)

- Lump due to an inflamed blocked meibomian gland duct, which will usually gradually resolve over a few weeks without treatment.
- Topical antibiotic ointment for 7–10 days.
- Incise and curette under a short general anaesthetic if not improving with treatment (see Chapter 26).

Molluscum contagiosum (Figure 25.3)

- Typically small, dome-shaped itchy lesions with central core of softer material.
- On hands, face and trunk and around eyes.
- Causes a follicular conjunctivitis.

Common oculo-orbital problems

- **Limbal dermoid** (Figure 25.4a): benign congenital tumour often associated with eyelid coloboma in Goldenhar's syndrome.
- **Dermoid cyst** (Figure 25.4b): smooth round non-tender immobile lump on orbital rim. Gradually grows. Risk of rupture. Contains cheesy white material +/− hairs.
- Dermolipoma (Figure 25.4c): benign congenital conjunctival and orbital yellow fatty lesion. Lies very close to lacrimal ductile openings, therefore advise caution in excision or leave. Risks a severe dry eye from lacrimal ductile damage.

Ptosis (drooping eyelid) (Figure 25.5)

- Congenital dystrophic (fatty levator muscle).
- Acquired third cranial nerve palsy (rare).
- Inflammation, such as vernal keratoconjunctivitis (Figure 25.5b).

Ptosis assessment

Measure the visual acuity, levator function, vertical palpebral aperture distance and skin crease height. Observe Bell's phenomenon. Look for aberrant eyelid movements with chewing and talking (Marcus Gunn jaw–winking ptosis).

Surgery

- Depends on the levator function.
- Very poor (<5 mm), internal suspension to the frontalis muscle (frontalis suspension).
- Good levator function from >5 mm up to 15 mm.
- Anterior or posterior approach levator resection (ALR or PLR, respectively).

There is a risk of amblyopia when the eyelid covers the pupil axis. Do an urgent frontalis suspension with non-autologous material (Gortex or Prolene) and later autogenous fascia lata frontalis suspension (where fascial strips are taken from their upper leg). If the eyelid is only slightly drooping and the child can easily 'see out from beneath it' by adopting a small chin-up head position, there is less risk of amblyopia. Wait until aged 4 years before ptosis surgery.

Sticky watering eyes

- A blocked nasolacrimal duct requires syringing and probing under endoscopic endonasal monitoring or dacryocystorhinostomy (DCR).
- Vernal and atopic conjunctivitis (Figure 25.5b): photophobia, swollen eyelids and itchy, stringy discharge that is worse in summer. History of atopy. Large giant papillae on tarsal conjunctiva and some small limbal lumps (limbal vernal). Treat with topical anti-inflammatory drops.
- Blepharitis: red-rimmed sticky eyes with a tendency to recurrent chalazia, blepharoconjunctivitis and watering. Treat by eyelid cleaning and topical antibiotic ointment.

Severe Orbital cellulitis (Figure 25.6)

Distinguish between pre-septal and post-septal orbital cellulitis when the child can be ill or febrile and requires admission.

Pre-septal cellulitis

- Involves only the eyelids but can spread posterior to the orbital septum to become post-septal.
- One or both eyelids are swollen and tender.
- Involves a white eye which moves fully with no impairment of vision or proptosis.
- Treat with intravenous (IV) antibiotics.

Post-septal cellulitis

- Potentially severe life-threatening condition (cavernous sinus thrombosis), unless treated.
- Painful orbital or eyelid red swelling and proptosis; child is feverish and unwell.
- Associated with an upper respiratory tract infection and undiagnosed sinusitis.
- May not be able to open eye to see limited eye movements.
- Conjunctiva red and swollen.
- Vision may be affected: reduced visual acuity and red desaturation with a relative afferent papillary defect due to optic nerve compression.
- Do a computed tomography scan to exclude sinus disease and subperiosteal abscess, which need surgical draining and bacteriology.
- Infection from *Haemophilus influenzae*, *Streptococcus* or *Staphylococcus* Gram-negative rods.
- Urgent admission, blood cultures and treatment with IV antibiotics.

Teenagers

Teenagers have their own visual problems with the onset of myopia, presentation of Leber's optic neuropathy, usually in the mid to late teens (see Chapter 53), 'hysterical' loss of vision, headaches and convergence insufficiency.

KEY POINTS

- Ptosis—risk of amblyopia when eyelid covers the visual axis.
- Ptosis—usually wait until 4 years of age before surgery is performed.
- Drain subperiosteal abscess in orbital cellulitis.

Figure 26.1 Cross-section of eyelid

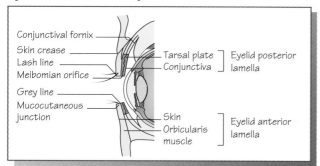

Conjunctival fornix
Skin crease
Lash line
Meibomian orifice
Grey line
Mucocutaneous junction

Tarsal plate
Conjunctiva
} Eyelid posterior lamella

Skin
Orbicularis muscle
} Eyelid anterior lamella

Figure 26.2 Meibomian glands and deeper layers of the eyelid

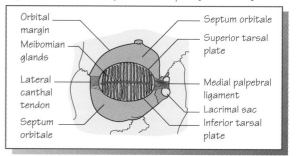

Orbital margin
Meibomian glands
Lateral canthal tendon
Septum orbitale

Septum orbitale
Superior tarsal plate
Medial palpebral ligament
Lacrimal sac
Inferior tarsal plate

Figure 26.3 Layers of the skin

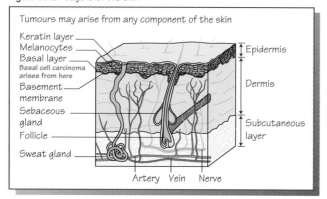

Tumours may arise from any component of the skin

Keratin layer
Melanocytes
Basal layer
Basal cell carcinoma arises from here
Basement membrane
Sebaceous gland
Follicle
Sweat gland

Epidermis
Dermis
Subcutaneous layer

Artery   Vein   Nerve

Figure 26.4 Diagram of a chalazion

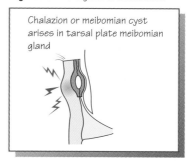

Chalazion or meibomian cyst arises in tarsal plate meibomian gland

Figure 26.5 How to evert the upper eyelid. (a) Patient looks down, (b) pull on the eyelashes and place a cotton bud above the skin crease and (c) evert

(a)
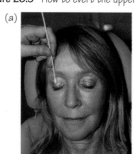

(b)
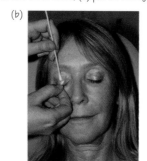

(c)
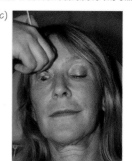

Figure 26.6 (a–d) Incision and curettage of a chalazion

(a)
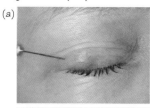

(b)
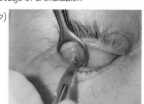

(c)
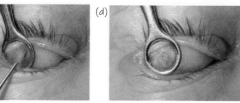

(d)

Figure 26.7 Basal cell carcinoma (BCC): right lower eyelid nodular BCC

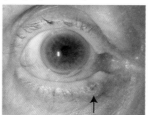

Figure 26.8 Squamous cell carcinoma (SCC): left lower eyelid SCC

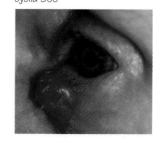

Ophthalmology at a Glance, Second Edition. Jane Olver, Lorraine Cassidy, Gurjeet Jutley, and Laura Crawley. © 2014 Jane Olver, Lorraine Cassidy, Gurjeet Jutley and Laura Crawley. Published 2014 by John Wiley & Sons, Ltd. Companion Website: www.ataglanceseries.com/ophthal

Eyelid lumps are common and include benign cysts and tumours as well as malignant skin and adnexal tumours. Tumours can arise from the skin, the deeper layers of the eyelid, the conjunctiva or the orbit (Figures 26.1, 26.2 and 26.3).

Aims

- Recognize a chalazion and understand its treatment.
- Recognize a basal cell carcinoma and distinguish it from a squamous cell carcinoma.
- Treat periocular basal cell carcinoma.

Differential diagnosis of periocular tumours

Many different lumps are found on the eyelids. An incision or excision biopsy is often required for histological analysis.

- Benign: chalazion, papilloma, retention cyst and sebaceous cyst.
- Malignant (in order of prevalence):
  - basal cell carcinoma (BCC)
  - squamous cell carcinoma (SCC)
  - sebaceous gland carcinoma (SGC)
  - malignant melanoma (MM)
  - Merkel cell tumour
  - other rare tumours (e.g. tumours of the sweat gland).

Benign lumps

Chalazion or meibomian cyst (Figure 26.4)

There are at least 27 meibomian glands in each eyelid. The meibomian glands secrete oil and if the oil becomes too thick, for instance in blepharitis and meibomianitis, a single duct can obstruct. Giant cells go in to try to remove the oil, but can accumulate and form a chalazion. The eyelid should be everted to see if there is a typical granuloma or grey appearance of the chalazion and to exclude other tumours (Figure 26.5).

A chalazion can be inflamed or quiet. Initial treatment of an inflamed chalazion is by hot compresses and topical antibiotic ointment four times a day for 2 weeks. If the lump persists as a quiet chalazion, surgical incision and curettage (I&C) is done (Figure 26.6).

How to do an I&C

- Local anaesthetic (topical plus infiltrative).
- Place a small eyelid clamp and evert the eyelid.
- Use an 11 blade to incise vertically into the cyst on the tarsal surface (in a direction away from the eye and avoiding the eyelid margin).
- Use a curette spoon to curette out the jelly.
- Place a firm pad plus chloromycetin ointment for up to 24 h.
- Continue the ointment three times a day for 4 days.

If an assumed chalazion recurs, particularly in an older person, do an incisional biopsy urgently for histopathological analysis as this may be a sebaceous gland carcinoma (meibomian gland carcinoma), a highly malignant tumour.

Solar keratosis (actinic keratosis)

These are dry scaly patches due to dysplastic intraepidermal proliferation of atypical keratinocytes, and they occur on the face in older, fair-skinned persons who have lived in sunny climates. There is a low risk of malignant transformation into SCC. Fortunately, many solar keratoses regress spontaneously over 1–2 years, but 15% recur. Treatment is with cryotherapy or 5-fluorouracil.

Malignant lumps

Basal cell carcinoma ('rodent ulcer') (Figure 26.7)

BCC is the commonest periocular malignant tumour. It occurs most frequently on the lower eyelid, the medial canthus, the upper lid and lastly the lateral canthus. It is typically a nodular pearly lump with no hair or lashes on it, with telangiectatic blood vessels. The central zone may bleed and ulcerate. It is usually nodular with distinct borders but can be morphoeic and have indistinct margins. BCC grows slowly by direct extension and destroys tissue locally. It can invade the orbit if neglected or inadequately treated. Early treatment is recommended by first doing an incisional biopsy to make the diagnosis and an excisional biopsy with a 2–4 mm margin of clear tissue or Mohs' micrographic surgery to completely remove the tumour.

BCC does not metastasize. After surgical excision there, the oculoplastic surgeon does the eyelid reconstruction. Cryotherapy and radiotherapy are occasional treatment options.

Mohs' micrographic surgery

Mohs' micrographic excision of BCC is a special technique to remove the BCC with frozen sections of the deep bed of the tumour to ensure complete excision. It is done by dermatological surgeons especially trained in the technique. It provides good clearance of tumour with maximum normal tissue preservation and low recurrence; therefore, it is ideal for the eyelids where complete tumour excision and tissue preservation for reconstruction are essential.

Mohs' micrographic excision is also used for SCC and meibomian cell carcinoma.

An oculoplastics-trained ophthalmologist does the periocular reconstruction after Mohs' micrographic excision.

Squamous cell carcinoma (Figure 26.8)

SCC is rarer than BCC but is more rapidly growing and has a greater potential for spread, especially perineurally. It is a red lump with a variable appearance. It is much more common in immunosuppressed patients, for instance post renal or liver transplant patients on long-term immunosuppression drugs.

Sebaceous gland carcinoma

SGC may masquerade as a recurrent chalazion or unilateral blepharitis in an elderly female patient. A large incisional biopsy is required for histopathologic analysis. This tumour can spread by lymphatics, and the patient requires radical neck excision. There is a significant 5-year mortality.

Malignant melanoma

Very rare but potentially very serious. Most pigmented lesions around the eye are benign, but the usual caveats apply—if there is an increase in size or if it bleeds, urgent referral is needed.

KEY POINTS

- A recurrent chalazion may not be a chalazion but a malignant tumour such as a sebaceous gland carcinoma.
- Basal cell carcinoma is the commonest eyelid malignancy.
- Mohs' micrographic surgery is the gold standard for excising periocular basal cell carcinoma.

Figure 27.1 Normal anterior eyelid anatomy

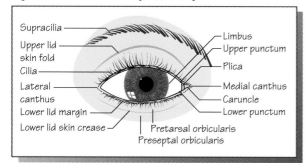

Supracilia
Upper lid skin fold
Cilia
Lateral canthus
Lower lid margin
Lower lid skin crease
Limbus
Upper punctum
Plica
Medial canthus
Caruncle
Lower punctum
Pretarsal orbicularis
Preseptal orbicularis

Figure 27.2 Cross section eyelid in orbit anatomy

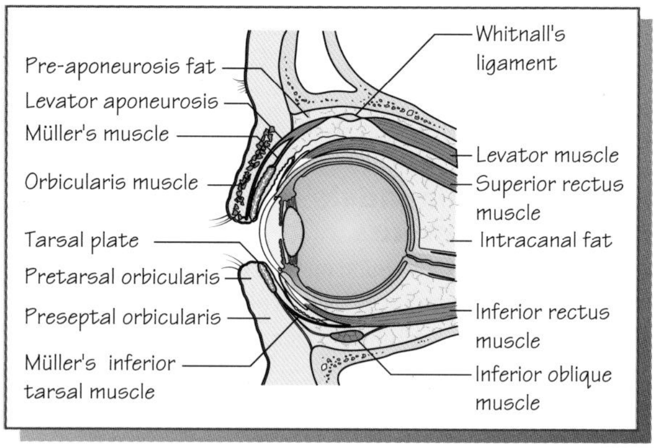

Pre-aponeurosis fat
Levator aponeurosis
Müller's muscle
Orbicularis muscle
Tarsal plate
Pretarsal orbicularis
Preseptal orbicularis
Müller's inferior tarsal muscle
Whitnall's ligament
Levator muscle
Superior rectus muscle
Intracanal fat
Inferior rectus muscle
Inferior oblique muscle

Nerve supply to eyelids

Upper eyelid
Levator palpebrae superioris (cranial nerve III) and Müller's superior tarsal muscle (sympathetic) open the upper eyelid
Orbicularis oculi (cranial nerve VII) closes the eyelid

Lower eyelid
The capsulopalpebral fascia (linked to the inferior rectus muscle – cranial nerve III) and Müller's lower tarsal muscle (sympathetic) help the lower lid move 2–4 mm downwards on downgaze and help open the lids
Orbicularis oculi (cranial nerve VII) closes the eyelid

Figure 27.3 Eyelid and brow measurements

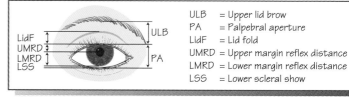

LidF
UMRD
LMRD
LSS
ULB
PA

ULB	= Upper lid brow
PA	= Palpebral aperture
LidF	= Lid fold
UMRD	= Upper margin reflex distance
LMRD	= Lower margin reflex distance
LSS	= Lower scleral show

KEY POINTS

- Measurement is important in eyelids
- Involutional entropion is treated temporarily with botulinum toxin A
- Facial palsy causes lagophthalmos and a risk of exposure keratitis

Eyelid malpositions

Figure 27.4 Congenital entropion – epiblepharon

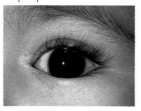

Figure 27.5 Involutional entropion

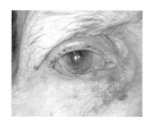

Figure 27.6 Distichiasis

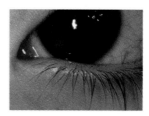

Definitions	
Trichiasis	= rubbing of abnormal inturned eyelashes against the eye causing discomfort
Distichiasis	= additional row of aberrant lashes arising from the meibomian orifices

Figure 27.7 Involutional ectropion

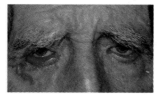

Bilateral tarsal aversion

Figure 27.8 Paralytic ectropion with lagophthalmos

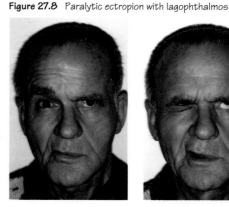

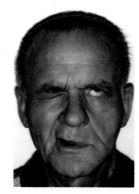

Left eye lagophalalmos due to orbitcularis oculi muscle weakness

Ophthalmology at a Glance, Second Edition. Jane Olver, Lorraine Cassidy, Gurjeet Jutley, and Laura Crawley. © 2014 Jane Olver, Lorraine Cassidy,
Gurjeet Jutley and Laura Crawley. Published 2014 by John Wiley & Sons, Ltd. Companion Website: www.ataglanceseries.com/ophthal

As patients age, you will find that the eyelids change position; they become more lax and turn inwards (entropion) or outwards (ectropion) or droop (ptosis). Occasionally with disease, an eyelid can also turn in, turn out, droop or even open more due to retraction.

Aims
• Examine an eyelid.
• Identify entropion (lid in) and ectropion (lid out).
• Identify ptosis (lid down) and eyelid retraction (lid up).

Eyelid anatomy
It is important to understand the bilaminar structure of the eyelids, which have an anterior lamella and a posterior lamella (Figures 27.1 and 27.2).

Eyelid function
The eyelids are mobile and serve to protect the eye and distribute the tears. They also contain the oily glands (meibomian glands) which produce the oil for the tear film. When assessing eyelid malposition, you have to observe and make measurements (Figure 27.3).

Eyelid examination
• Measure visual acuity!
• Look at the whole face, eyebrow height and symmetry.
• Measure the vertical palpebral aperture (PA) and margin reflex distances (MRDs) and the amount of scleral show (SS) above or below the limbus in millimetres.
• Measure the levator function (LF) in millimetres—upper-lid excursion from full downgaze to full upgaze.
• Assess the orbicularis strength and Bell's phenomenon (do the eyes roll upwards under upper eyelid on closure?).
• Exclude aberrant eyelid movements.
• Lag on downgaze—eyelid hangs up on downgaze.
• Detect lagophthalmos—eye remains partially open on attempted closure.
• Exclude distichiasis, trichiasis, entropion and ectropion.
• Examine tarsal conjunctiva and conjunctival fornices to exclude scar or tumour.

Eyelid malpositions
Entropion (see Figures 27.4 and 27.5)
In entropion, the eyelid turns in towards the cornea and the lashes touch the surface of the eye. Another cause of eyelashes touching the eye is distichiasis, where an aberrant row of eyelashes arises from the meibomian orifices with the eyelid margin in a normal position (Figure 27.6).
Aetiology
• Involutional—older persons.
• Spastic (causes by severe squeezing of the eyelids in response to ocular discomfort).
• Cicatricial entropion secondary to conjunctival scarring, such as staphylococcal lid margin disease (mild entropion), ocular cicatricial pemphigoid (severe entropion) or trachoma.
Pathogenesis
Thinning of the lamellae and disinsertion of the lower lid retractors. The pre-septal overrides the pretarsal orbicularis, causing in-turning of the lower lid.
Symptoms
Ocular irritation, discomfort, reflex watering (hypersecretion), redness and occasionally keratitis if left untreated. It is worse when lying down (e.g. reading in bed).

Treatment
• Temporary treatment: lid taping and topical lubricants; botulinum toxin A injected into the pre-septal orbicularis alleviates symptoms for up to 4 months but has to be repeated.
• Surgery is the mainstay of treatment.
• Lateral tarsal strip with everting sutures (LTS + ES). This shortens the lower eyelid horizontally and everts the eyelid.
• Simple everting sutures (ES) alone.

Ectropion (Figure 27.7)
In ectropion, the lower eyelid turns outwards away from the eye.
Aetiology
• Involutional—older persons.
• Cicatricial causes (e.g. post blepharoplasty, actinic, following skin tumour excision or from contact dermatitis).
• Mechanical—the weight of an eyelid tumour pulling the eyelid outwards.
• Facial palsy—paralytic (seventh cranial nerve (CN) palsy) (Figure 27.8).
Symptoms
Watering, irritation, grittiness and redness.
Treatment
• Involutional ectropion—shorten the eyelid horizontally and turn the medial part inwards using a lateral tarsal strip and excision of a diamond shape of medial tarsal conjunctiva or medial spindle (LTS + MS).
• Cicatricial ectropion—skin graft or flap to lengthen the anterior lamella; horizontal shortening may also be required.
• Contact dermatitis—stop the causative eye drops or change to preservative-free drops. No surgery needed.
• For facial palsy (see Chapter 30).

Ptosis
Eyelid ptosis is abnormally low position of the upper eyelid margin.
Congenital paediatric ptosis (see Chapter 25)
Aetiology
• Involutional or aponeurotic (thinning or dehiscence of the anterior part of the levator, the aponeurosis): good levator function (LF). Occurs commonly in the elderly and with contact lens wear.
• Myogenic: LF is very poor. Includes the congenital dystrophic (fatty) levator muscles in children and myopathies in adults (e.g. chronic progressive external ophthalmoplegia).
• Neurogenic: the LF is usually poor (e.g. third CN palsy).
• Mechanical: usually good LF (e.g. neurofibromatosis).
• Traumatic ptosis may be aponeurotic, myogenic or neurogenic.
Symptoms
• Cosmetically poor appearance
• Functional—reduces the visual field.
Management Depends on the type of ptosis and LF.
• Normal or good LF is >10 mm, moderate LF is 5–10 mm and poor LF is <5 mm.
• Good and moderate LF: anterior levator resection (ALR)—tuck or advance the levator aponeurosis or muscle.
• Poor LF: frontalis suspension with autogenous fascia lata.
Eyelid retraction
Lower motor neurone facial palsy (seventh CN palsy) and thyroid eye disease can both cause exposure keratitis. See Chapters 30 and 54.

28 Lacrimation (tearing)

Figure 28.1 Lacrimal anatomy

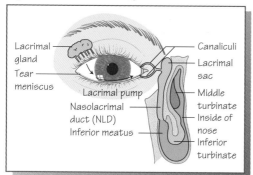

Lacrimal gland
Tear meniscus
Lacrimal pump
Nasolacrimal duct (NLD)
Inferior meatus
Canaliculi
Lacrimal sac
Middle turbinate
Inside of nose
Inferior turbinate

Figure 28.2 Blocked nasolacrimal duct

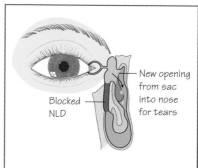

Blocked NLD
New opening from sac into nose for tears

Figure 28.3 Dacryocystorhinostomy (DCR)

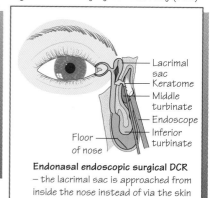

Lacrimal sac
Keratome
Middle turbinate
Endoscope
Inferior turbinate
Floor of nose

Endonasal endoscopic surgical DCR – the lacrimal sac is approached from inside the nose instead of via the skin

Figure 28.4 Mucocoele
Right mucocoele–chronic dacryocystitis

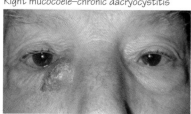

Figure 28.5 Lacrimal irrigation. (a) Syringing and (b) probing

(a)
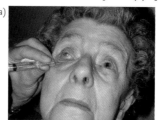

(b)
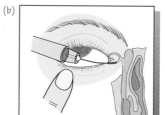

Figure 28.6 Nasal endoscopy

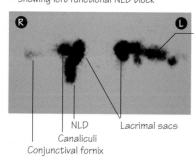

This is a very useful technique that provides direct observation of the nasal space both in out-patients and during lacrimal surgery. A rigid Hopkins 4 mm 0° rigid nasal endoscope is used to look at the opening of the NLD into the nose and at the DCR surgery site

Figure 28.7 Normal dacryocystography (DCG): the left side shows free drainage contrast media into nose

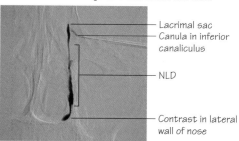

Lacrimal sac
Canula in inferior canaliculus
NLD
Contrast in lateral wall of nose

Figure 28.8 Nuclear lacrimal scintigraphy – showing left functional NLD block

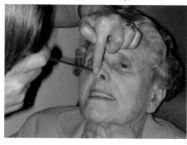

R   L

Pooling of tears containing technetium 99 in the conjunctival fornix

NLD
Canaliculi
Lacrimal sacs
Conjunctival fornix

Figure 28.9 Left external skin approach dacryocystorhinostomy (DCR) – surgery view

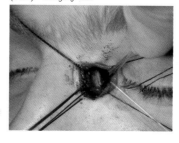

A mucosal-lined opening is made from the lacrimal sac to the nose after the intervening bone has been removed

Figure 28.10 Functioning DCR ostium. Fluorescein passing freely down the lateral wall of the nose

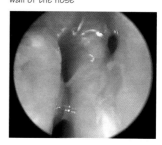

Watering eyes occur when there are too many tears or poor tear drainage.

Lacrimal anatomy and physiology (Figure 28.1)
Lacrimal anatomy
The lacrimal drainage system consists of the punta, canaliculi, lacrimal sac and nasolacrimal duct (NLD).

Lacrimal physiology
The tears are produced by the lacrimal gland and the accessory lacrimal tissue (the glands of Krause and Wolfring) and are swept over the eye surface with each blink. Tear evaporation occurs (approximately 25%). The marginal tear strip drains via the lower canaliculus predominantly (70%) and 30% via the upper canaliculus. The lacrimal pump mechanism is the action of the eyelids contracting and pumping the tears into the lacrimal sac.

Aims
- Understanding the difference between hypersecretion and epiphora.
- Using syringing in assessment of epiphora.
- Dacryocystorhinostomy.

Nasolacrimal duct obstruction is a common cause of epiphora (watering eye; Figure 28.2). Surgery to correct this is called dacryocystorhinostomy (DCR) in which an opening between the lacrimal sac and the nose is made (Figure 28.3).

DCR is done via the nose (endonasal) or via the skin (external approach).

Watering eyes
There are many causes of a watering eye, and careful assessment is required.
- Hypersecretion: excess production of tears in response to stimulation of the trigeminal nerve from corneal irritation (e.g. a corneal foreign body), dry eye or conjunctival irritation (e.g. blepharitis or conjunctivitis).
- Epiphora: reduced tear drainage from lacrimal system obstruction at any point from the punctum, canaliculus, sac or nasolacrimal duct. Nasolacrimal duct obstruction is the commonest cause.

The commonest cause of epiphora is a blocked nasolacrimal duct (NLD). This can be primary from chronic inflammation with subsequent fibrosis and stenosis, or, less commonly, secondary from sarcoidosis, Wegener's granulomatosis, tumour or trauma.

DCR is the treatment of choice.

Mucocoele (see Figure 28.4)
A mucocoele is a dilated lacrimal sac containing mucous. It is often seen as a lump at the medial canthus, and it is caused when the nasolacrimal duct distal to it is blocked.

Functional epiphora: epiphora in the presence of patent syringing without hypersecretion due to:
- eyelid malposition (e.g. lower lid ectropion)
- lacrimal pump failure (e.g. facial palsy)

- punctual, canalicular and nasolacrimal duct stenosis (without a complete obstruction).

Investigation of a watering eye
History
Stickiness or worse watering occurs outside or constantly. Often patient has a history of nasal disease, sinusitis, polyps or nasal trauma, previous conjunctivitis, eye drops and/or drugs.

Assessment of the watering eye
- External examination of the forehead and the periocular and medial canthus is performed to exclude eyelid malposition and mucocoele.
- Fluorescein dye retention test: watch a drop of fluorescein 2% rapidly disappear from the conjunctiva if the system is patent or show dye retention if it is blocked.
- Slit lamp examination can do the following:
  - Exclude blepharitis.
  - Exclude punctual stenosis.
  - Determine tear meniscus height.
- Probe and then syringe and irrigate the lacrimal system with saline (Figure 28.5).
- Nasal endoscopy (Figure 28.6)
  - The nasal endoscope is used to look inside the nasal space to exclude nasal pathology such as tumours, inflammation and polyps as well as anatomical variations.
- Radiology imaging studies
  - Dacryocystography (DCG) with radio-opaque material for anatomical detail (Figure 28.7) is used to determine the site of the obstruction.
  - Lacrimal scintigraphy is a nuclear scanning technique using a drop of technetium 99 placed in the conjunctival fornix and a gamma camera to observe its passive drainage (Figure 28.8).
  - It is used to detect physiological tear drainage in the assessment of functional NLD obstruction with partial obstruction.

Surgery
DCR can be external (via the skin) or endonasal (via the nose).
- Aim of DCR: create a functioning rhinostomy between the lacrimal sac and the nasal space.
- External (skin incision) approach.
- Endonasal DCR (via the nose) is less invasive (Figure 28.9). The rigid nasal endoscope provides good illumination and magnification transnasally. Many patients prefer endonasal DCR because it avoids a skin incision. Figure 28.10 shows a functioning DCR ostium in the nose.

KEY POINTS

- Ectropion is a cause of epiphora.
- Endoscopic endonasal DCR avoids a skin incision.
- External approach DCR still has the best results—95–98% success.

Figure 29.1 Cross-section of the globe and orbit

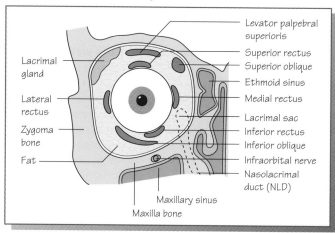

Levator palpebral superioris
Superior rectus
Superior oblique
Ethmoid sinus
Medial rectus
Lacrimal sac
Inferior rectus
Inferior oblique
Infraorbital nerve
Nasolacrimal duct (NLD)
Maxillary sinus
Maxilla bone
Lacrimal gland
Lateral rectus
Zygoma bone
Fat

Figure 29.2 Axial view of the orbit

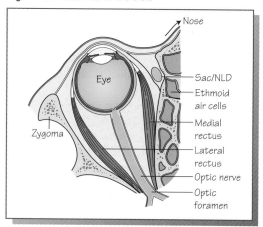

Nose
Eye
Sac/NLD
Ethmoid air cells
Medial rectus
Lateral rectus
Optic nerve
Optic foramen
Zygoma

Figure 29.3 Bony orbital walls

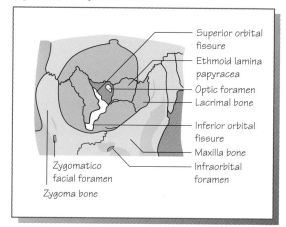

Superior orbital fissure
Ethmoid lamina papyracea
Optic foramen
Lacrimal bone
Inferior orbital fissure
Maxilla bone
Infraorbital foramen
Zygomatico facial foramen
Zygoma bone

Measurement of exophthalmos (proptosis)/enophthalmos

Figure 29.4 (a) Hertel measurement of eye protrusion or the degree to which eyes are sunken in and (b) a close-up of Hertel measurement

(a)
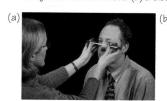

(b)
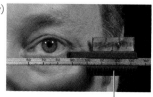

Blue triangle lined up with marker line
This patient measures 21 mm at 100 mm

Radiological imaging

Figure 29.5 (a) Left post-septal orbital cellulitis with proptosis, eye closed and limited eye movements and (b) computed tomography scan showing sinus disease and a subperiosteal orbital abscess

(a)
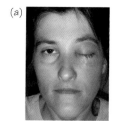

(b)
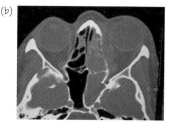

The orbit is a space: the eye, eye muscles, fat, nerves, vessels and optic nerve are all enclosed on four sides by the bony orbit.

This chapter covers the anatomy of the orbit and the systematic approach to examining a patient with proptosis. The most common cause of proptosis in adult patients is thyroid eye disease, also known as Graves' orbitopathy.

Aims
- Assessment of a patient with proptosis.
- Orbital imaging techniques.
- Differential diagnosis of proptosis.

Orbital anatomy (Figures 29.1, 29.2 and 29.3)
The bony orbit has four margins anterior and four walls. It lies adjacent to the ethmoid sinus (medial) and maxillary sinus (inferior). It contains the optic foramen for the optic nerve and ophthalmic artery, the superior orbital fissure (cranial nerves and blood vessels) and the inferior orbital fissure. The infraorbital nerve lies in the floor, partly in a bony canal. The orbit contains a lot of fat and connective tissue septae that support and cushion the eye and its muscles, optic nerve, nerves and blood vessels.

Orbital terms
- Proptosis: eye protrudes forwards out of orbit; also called exophthalmos.
- Enophthalmos: eye is sunken into orbit.
- Anophthalmia: socket contains no eye.
- Pseudophthalmia: socket contains an orbital implant.
- Microphthalmia: socket contains a very small eye or ocular remnant.
- Phthisical eye: a blind shrunken eye.

Loss of an eye
- Enucleation: removal of an eye in its entirety—detaching it from the optic nerve and the extraocular muscles.
- Evisceration: removal of the contents of the eye, leaving the outer sclera, the attached optic nerve and extraocular muscles.
- Post-enucleation socket syndrome: deep sunken 'eye' when the volume of the removed eye has not been adequately replaced.
- Prosthetic eye: artificial eye, usually made of acrylic.

Expansion of the orbital space
Orbital decompression is removing (usually) the medial and lateral orbital walls to expand the orbit in thyroid eye disease.

Orbital assessment
History
- Gradual or sudden onset. If slow and non-inflamed, it is more likely to be benign.
- Unilateral or bilateral.
- Orbital swelling, or sunken.
- Orbital pain.
- Periorbital redness (e.g. orbital cellulitis).
- Periorbital numbness.
- Visual disturbance.
- Double vision.
- Drooping eyelid.
- Systemic: malignancy or thyroid problem.
- Previous trauma.
- An asculation for a bruit is a caroticocavernous fistula.

Clinical examination
Visual function (if eye is present) and eye examination
- Visual acuity and pupil reactions.
- Colour vision ± visual fields.
- Retina and optic disc.

Globe position
Measure proptosis with Hertel exophthalmometry (Figure 29.4)—is it axial or non-axial?

Measure proptosis or enophthalmos (Figure 29.4)
Assess type of proptosis:
- Axial proptosis (anteroposterior protruding globe) without horizontal or vertical displacement. This suggests a generalized orbitopathy such as thyroid eye disease or an intraconal mass.
- Non-axial proptosis. Horizontal or vertical displacement of the globe is caused by a mass pushing it sideways. For instance, a lacrimal gland tumour in the superolateral quadrant pushes the globe inferomedially.

Assess enophthalmos
- Is there a history of trauma and possible orbital floor fracture?
- Is there a phthisical eye?
- Is there an ocular prosthesis?
- Has the patient had an eye enucleated?
- Was there an orbital implant placed after enucleation or evisceration?
- Is there a secondary post-enucleation socket syndrome?
- Are the eye movements restricted? Is the socket lining contracted?

Check the cranial nerve (CN) function
- Third, fourth and sixth CN: extraocular muscle movement.
- Seventh CN: upper facial musculature.
- Fifth CN: corneal, periorbital and forehead sensation.

Feel the orbit
Palpate the orbital rim. If a mass is detected, is it separate from the rim? Describe its feel and shape, and draw a picture of its shape and location.

Complete the examination
Palpate the temporal fossa for extension of swelling. Exclude preauricular, submandibular and cervical lymphadenopathy. Examine the neck for thyroid enlargement or thyroid scar. Check sensation in the skin around the orbit.

Investigations
- Computed tomography scanning (Figure 29.5): axial and coronal views show the position of the optic nerve well, and also the sinuses and orbital walls (request bone window settings, too). Suspected vascular lesions need contrast.
- Magnetic resonance imaging: good for soft tissue but does not show bone as well.
- Orbital ultrasound: colour Doppler ultrasound to measure size and show blood flow and velocity within lesion.

> **KEY POINTS**
> - Proptosis is axial or non-axial.
> - Palpate the orbit to help detect a mass.

Figure 30.1 *Graves' orbitopathy (thyroid eye disease). (a) and (b) Marked proptosis and redness—active phase and (c) computed tomography (CT) scan – enlarged medial and inferior rectus muscles in Graves' orbitopathy*

(a) 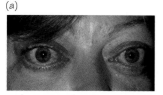 (b)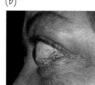

(c)

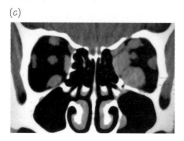

Figure 30.2 *(a) and (b) Bilateral proptosis, periorbital swelling and left esotropia—quiet phase*

(a) 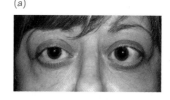 (b)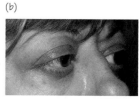

Figure 30.3 *Tumour behind eye. (a) Right proptosis from large cavernous haemangioma and (b) CT scan showing tumour (benign)*

(a) 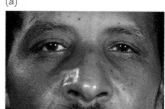 (b)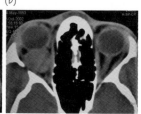

Figure 30.5 *Enucleation. Indications for enucleation include a painful blind eye, choroidal malignant melanoma and a severely disrupted eye following trauma. The eye is eviscerated if there is an intractable endophthalmitis. Post-enucleation socket syndrome; no orbital implant is placed at time of enucleation. (a) Wearing a thick artificial eye but still very enophthalmic and (b) a thick artificial eye*

(a) 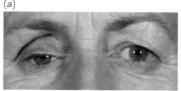 (b)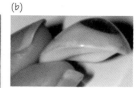

Figure 30.4 *Chronic facial palsy*

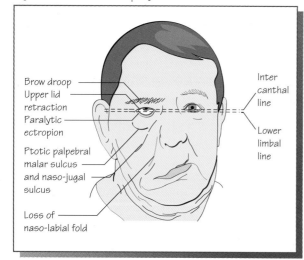

- Brow droop
- Upper lid retraction
- Paralytic ectropion
- Ptotic palpebral malar sulcus and naso-jugal sulcus
- Loss of naso-labial fold
- Inter canthal line
- Lower limbal line

Figure 30.6 *Porous polyethylene sphere implant inserted into socket. Orbital sphere implant is needed to replace lost volume*

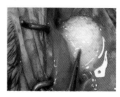

Graves' orbitopathy and facial palsy are common problems managed by the oculoplastic surgeon in conjunction with the endocrinologist, neurologist, neurosurgeon and plastic surgeon. The aim of the oculoplastic surgeon is to ensure that the patient maintains good vision, a comfortable eye and surgically rehabilitates.

Orbital tumours are a rare cause of proptosis.

Aims

- Manage Graves' orbitopathy.
- Manage facial palsy.
- Differential diagnosis of orbital proptosis.

Common orbital problems

- Adult:
  - Graves' orbitopathy (thyroid eye disease) (most common)
  - idiopathic orbital inflammation
  - cavernous haemangioma
  - lacrimal gland tumour
  - secondary tumours
  - nerve cell or sheath tumours.
- Child:
  - dermoid cyst
  - haemangioma

Ophthalmology at a Glance, Second Edition. Jane Olver, Lorraine Cassidy, Gurjeet Jutley, and Laura Crawley. © 2014 Jane Olver, Lorraine Cassidy, Gurjeet Jutley and Laura Crawley. Published 2014 by John Wiley & Sons, Ltd. Companion Website: www.ataglanceseries.com/ophthal

- rhabdomyosarcoma
- craniofacial abnormality.

Graves' ophthalmopathy (Figures 30.1 and 30.2)

This is also known as thyroid eye disease, dysthyroid eye disease, Graves' orbitopathy and Von Below disease.

Patients with Graves' ophthalmopathy usually develop their exophthalmos within 6–12 months of becoming hyperthyroid. Male patients and smokers have a more aggressive disease.

There is an active phase with inflammation which lasts up to 1 year (Figure 30.1a), and a subsequent inactive stable phase (Figure 30.2). During the active phase there is increased fibrosis of the muscles and fat, contributing to the signs and symptoms of exophthalmos, eyelid retraction and restricted eye movement. The active phase is treated medically with immunosuppression (e.g. steroids and azathioprine). Once the disease is inactive, surgery to the orbit, muscles and eyelids can be considered.

> **WARNING**
>
> ▶ Early orbital decompression surgery is done only if there is marked compressive optic neuropathy.

There is a varied presentation:
- Proptosis.
- Reduced colour vision from optic nerve compression.
- Restrictive strabismus with mainly inferior and/or medial rectus muscle enlargement causing diplopia.
- Eyelid retraction.
- Lagophthalmos.
- Exposure keratitis.
- Conjunctival redness and cheimosis.
- Periorbital swelling.

The aim of treatment is to preserve vision, with eyes comfortable and looking normal, with full lid closure.

Orbital and lacrimal gland tumours
(Figure 30.3)

Orbital and lacrimal gland tumours cause proptosis and require incisional or excisional biopsy by a trained oculoplastics orbital surgeon. Lymphoma and metastases are the commonest malignant tumours.

Many anterior and mid-orbital tumours can be biopsied via a skin approach. More posterior intraconal and lacrimal gland tumours (pleomorphic adenoma) may require excision via a lateral orbitotomy.

Facial palsy (Figure 30.4)

This is caused by Bell's palsy, herpes virus or posterior fossa tumour (sphenoidal meningioma).

The eye symptoms include:
- lagophthalmos (inability to close the eye fully)
- tearing
- red sore eye
- exposure keratitis
- reduced visual acuity
- brow ptosis
- upper eyelid ptosis
- lower eyelid paralytic ectropion
- cheek ptosis.

Management is initially to preserve vision and keep the eye comfortable, and it is followed by surgical oculoplastic rehabilitation.

Table 30.1 Graves' orbitopathy management

Indication	Phase	Medical treatment	Surgery
Compressive optic neuropathy	Active therapy	• Pulsed steroid decompression • Systemic steroids, azathioprine and orbital radiotherapy	Orbital
Proptosis	Inactive		Orbital decompression
Strabismus	Inactive		Adjustable suture rectus recession
Eyelid retraction	Inactive		• Graduated retractor recession (upper eyelids) • Hard palate mucosal graft, alloderm or auricular cartilage (lower eyelids)
Periorbital swelling	Inactive		Blepharoplasty
Skin changes	Inactive		Laser resurfacing skin

Treatment: Lubricant drops and ointment, punctual plugs, lower eyelid horizontal tightening, insertion upper eyelid gold weights, lower upper eyelid, cheek lift and hyaluronic acid gel cheek volumization.

Removal of an eye—enucleation and evisceration (Figure 30.5)

Enucleation is done if there is severe ocular trauma which cannot be salvaged, for painful blind eye and for large intra-ocular tumour (e.g. malignant melanoma) where there is no other treatment option.

Evisceration is done if there is endophthalmitis and the walls of the eye can be preserved. The intraocular contents including the lens, vitreous, retina and choroid are removed as well as the cornea.

When an eye is removed by enucleation or its contents removed by evisceration, its volume must be replaced in order to avoid a sunken orbital appearance.

A buried spherical orbital implant (Figure 30.6) is inserted to which the rectus muscles are attached either directly or indirectly via a cover material. An ocular prosthesis (artificial eye) is then made to match the normal eye; usually it is acrylic and hand painted (Figure 30.5b).

If the volume of the enucleated or eviscerated eye is not replaced, the patient has a sunken socket appearance called post-enucleation socket syndrome and will need a secondary buried orbital implant.

> **KEY POINTS**
>
> • Graves' orbitopathy—do decompression before eyelid surgery.
> • Monitor the vision carefully in facial palsy, and protect the vision and keep the eye comfortable.
> • It is important to replace the eye volume lost at enucleation or evisceration with an orbital implant or artificial eye.

Figure 31.1 Fundus photograph of a flat, pigmented choroidal naevus. Note the presence of drusen and retinal pigment epithelial changes, which implies chronicity

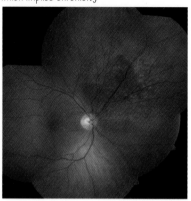

Figure 31.2 Fundus photograph of a pigmented choroidal melanoma.. Note the elevated 'collar stud'-shaped lesion

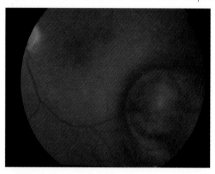

Figure 31.4 Fundus photo of a retinal capillary haemangioma. Note the large feeder vessel

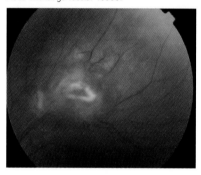

Figure 31.3 Leukocoria (white reflex) from the left eye. Causes of leukocoria include retinoblastoma

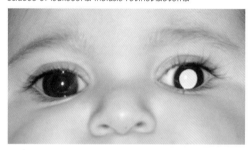

Figure 31.5 Fundus photograph of a circumscribed choroidal haemangioma above the optic nerve. Note the classic orange color of the lesion

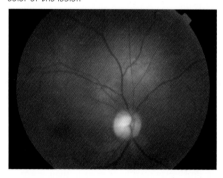

Figure 31.6 Slit lamp photograph of a conjunctival squamous cell neoplasia. Note the classic gelatinous, nodular conjunctival lesion

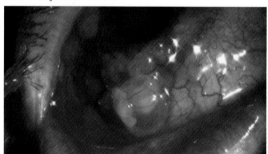

Figure 31.7 Slit lamp photograph of a conjunctival melanoma

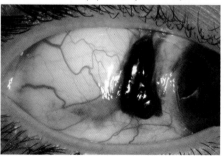

KEY POINTS

- The commonest primary fundus tumour of adults is the benign choroidal naevus. Its risk of transformation to melanoma is low
- Choroidal malignant melanoma is rare and can present with a retinal detachment or be totally asymptomatic
- Retinoblastoma is the most common childhood intraocular cancer. Any child with a white pupillary reflex requires a fundus examination to rule out retinoblastoma

Introduction

Neoplasia of the eye, although uncommon, can be devastating, as some tumours are not only sight threatening but also life threatening. Ophthalmologists with an interest in ocular oncology manage cancers of the eye and adnexae. Benign and malignant tumours affect the eye, including naevus, melanoma, haemangioma, metastasis, retinoblastoma, lymphoma, astrocytoma, osteoma as well as others. Pattern recognition is important, as biopsy for diagnosis is performed rarely and in some cases, such as retinoblastoma, it is contraindicated due to risk of tumour seeding.

Choroidal naevus

The commonest fundus tumour is a benign naevus, which arises from melanocytes of the choroidal stroma; it is often discovered as an incidental finding and is rarely symptomatic. It is a flat or minimally elevated grey, dark or sometimes pale lesion (Figure 31.1). Overlying changes such as drusen or retinal pigment epithelial changes imply chronicity. Subretinal fluid, lipofuscin and growth raise the suspicion for malignancy (melanoma). Approximately 10% of the white population has a choroidal naevus, and the risk of malignant transformation is low.

Choroidal melanoma

The most common primary malignant tumour of the posterior uvea (choroid and ciliary body) is melanoma (Figure 31.2). Symptoms include blurred vision and flashing lights (photopsiae), depending on the size and location of the tumour, but they are frequently asymptomatic and found on routine check by an optometrist. Very large melanomas can present with a painful blind eye from neovascular glaucoma. Any retinal detachment should have a careful fundus check to rule out the presence of a tumour. The incidence of uveal melanoma is 6 cases per million people.

Examination reveals a dome-shaped or 'collar stud' mass which is located in the choroid (deep to the retina) and usually pigmented, but can occasionally be partly or entirely non-pigmented (amelanotic). Retinal detachment and lipofuscin deposition are common features.

Management options include charged particle irradiation, plaque brachytherapy, local resection, enucleation, laser treatment or rarely observation. Deciding on which treatment modality should be employed depends on multiple factors including the tumour size, visual acuity of the affected eye and contralateral eye, age and general health of the patient and presence of metastases. Metastatic spread at the time of treatment is unusual, but systemic screening is advised for detection of liver involvement, even years after treatment of the ocular primary.

Retinoblastoma

Retinoblastoma is the most common intraocular malignancy of childhood, and its incidence is 1 in 15 000 live births. It can be unilateral or bilateral, and the overall mean age at diagnosis is 18 months. The most common and best known initial clinical sign is a white pupillary reflex, called leukocoria (Figure 31.3), but other presentations include a squint, raised intraocular pressure and orbital cellulitis. It is known to have one of the best cure rates (>95%) of all childhood cancers in the developed world.

There are two forms of the disease: a heritable (40%) and non-heritable form (60%). Also, two-thirds of the cases are unilateral, and the other third are bilateral. The retinoblastoma gene, Rb1 (chromosome 13), is a tumour suppressor, and both alleles need to have the mutation for retinoblastoma to manifest (Knudson's double-hit hypothesis). If both mutations are in somatic cells, this is the non-heritable form and these cases are unifocal and unilateral. If one mutation occurs in a germ line cell, then one somatic mutation in a retinal progenitor cell results in usually multifocal, bilateral tumours that present earlier. These patients have a cancer syndrome, and once they survive retinoblastoma, they are prone to develop systemic cancers such as osteosarcoma and melanoma.

Retinoblastomas usually begin as small, transparent retinal tumours. As they enlarge, they become white, opaque and calcified. Tumours can grow into the vitreous cavity (endophytic), under the retina (exophytic) or both. The management of retinoblastoma is complex. Options include chemotherapy, cryotherapy, laser photocoagulation, thermotherapy and enucleation.

Vascular tumours

Vascular tumours include haemangiomas of the choroid or retina, they and are benign. Retinal capillary haemangiomas (Figure 31.4) are associated with von Hippel–Lindau syndrome. Choroidal haemangiomas that are circumscribed are non-syndromic (Figure 31.5), but diffuse ones are a feature of Sturge–Weber syndrome. Treatment modalities for haemangiomas are designed to reduce leakage and preserve vision, and these include laser photocoagulation, photodynamic therapy and external beam radiotherapy.

Ocular metastasis

Secondary deposits occur in the eye, particularly in the choroid due to its vascular nature. These present as yellow creamy subretinal deposits that grow rapidly, and in two-thirds of cases the primary site is already known. Staging investigations may reveal intracranial metastases. Treatment involves controlling the primary tumour site, and also local treatment to the eye with external beam radiotherapy or photodynamic therapy to try to preserve as much vision as possible. The commonest primary sites are lung in men and breast in women.

Conjunctival squamous cell carcinoma (SCC)

SCC is the most common malignancy of the conjunctiva, and its incidence is about 1 to 2.8 per 100 000 people per year. Chronic sun exposure and immunosuppression are risk factors. Presentation is with red eye, pain, watering, burning and decreased vision. The appearance is of gelatinous, papillary, leukoplakic, diffuse or nodular lesions on the conjunctiva (Figure 31.6). Treatment is by excision and cryotherapy. Adjuvant treatments include radiotherapy and topical chemotherapy agents.

Conjunctival melanoma

This arises most commonly from primary acquired conjunctival melanosis with cancer predisposing atypical cells, but it can arise from a naevus or de novo (Figure 31.7). Most cases occur in patients in their seventh decade, and they are managed with excision and cryotherapy. Adjuvant treatments include radiotherapy and topical chemotherapy. Distant metastasis can occur, and involvement of the orbit requires exenteration.

Conclusion

Ocular oncology is an important branch of ophthalmology as many of these patients have diseases that carry significant morbidity and mortality. Pattern recognition of clinical signs that point towards malignancy is imperative.

Figure 32.1 Anatomy of the external eye and the lid margin zone (inset)

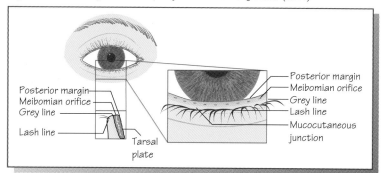

Posterior margin
Meibomian orifice
Grey line
Lash line

Tarsal plate

Posterior margin
Meibomian orifice
Grey line
Lash line
Mucocutaneous junction

Figure 32.2 Tear film

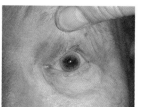

Lipid layer

Aqueous layer

Mucin

Corneal epithelial cells (microvilli)

Figure 32.3 Blepharitis

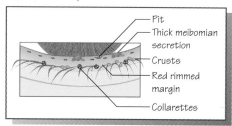

Pit
Thick meibomian secretion
Crusts
Red rimmed margin
Collarettes

Figure 32.4 Acne rosacea

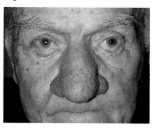

Figure 32.6 Pterygium

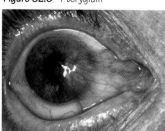

Figure 32.5 Upper eyelid entropion. (a) Mild cicatricial from chronic staphylococcal lid margin disease, (b everted upper eyelid, (c) lateral view showing eyelashes touching the cornea

(a)

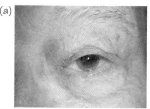

(b)

Everted upper eyelid
Linear scarring
Tarsal conjunctiva

(c)

Conjunctiva
Scarring
Cornea
Posterior marginization of meibomian orifice and blunting of posterior margin

Figure 32.7 Superior limbic keratitis

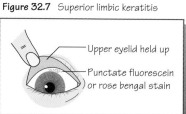

Upper eyelid held up

Punctate fluorescein or rose bengal stain

Figure 32.8 Ocular cicatricial pemphigoid

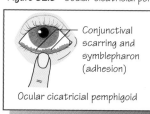

Conjunctival scarring and symblepharon (adhesion)

Ocular cicatricial pemphigoid

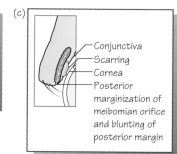

Ophthalmology at a Glance, Second Edition. Jane Olver, Lorraine Cassidy, Gurjeet Jutley, and Laura Crawley. © 2014 Jane Olver, Lorraine Cassidy, Gurjeet Jutley and Laura Crawley. Published 2014 by John Wiley & Sons, Ltd. Companion Website: www.ataglanceseries.com/ophthal

You should recognize and treat blepharitis, meibomian gland dysfunction and dry eyes which are the most common causes of ocular discomfort in adult patients.

Aims

Detection and medical management of:

- Blepharitis and meibomian gland dysfunction (MGD).
- Dry eyes.
- Allergic eye disease.

The tear film

The eyelid margins have lashes on the anterior lamella, and the meibomian orifices open behind the grey line from the posterior lamella (Figure 32.1). The tear film is bound to the cornea by microvilli glycocalyx on the epithelial goblet cells. The deepest layer is mucin, which is very thin; the middle layer is aqueous and the surface layer is lipid, from the meibomian glands (Figure 32.2).

Diseases of the external eye

- Blepharitis and meibomian gland dysfunction (MGD)
- Trachoma causing cicatricial entropion
- Pterygium
- Allergic eye disease.

Diseases primarily affecting the tear film, epithelium and conjunctiva

- Idiopathic dry eye
- Severe dry eye: Sjögren's syndrome and other autoimmune conditions
- Graft versus host disease
- Stevens–Johnson syndrome
- Ocular cicatricial pemphigoid.

Treatment

Depends on the underlying cause. If severe, corneal scarring with superficial vascularization leads to reduced vision and even corneal perforation.

Common conditions

Blepharitis and meibomian gland dysfunction (MGD)

Blepharitis

Low-grade chronic staphylococcal lid margin disease with 'red-rimmed' eyelids in young adults and middle-aged persons (Figure 32.3).

Symptoms: itchy, sore, watery eyes.

Signs: red-rimmed lid margins, eyelash crusts and collarettes, and distorted lid margin microanatomy (irregularities, pits and telangiectasia).

Management: Blepharitis cannot be 'cured' but can be managed to minimize symptoms, which are often a nuisance but rarely sight threatening. Daily lid hygiene is imperative.

- Warm compresses twice daily. Run a flannel under warm tap water, and apply to the closed eyelids for 1 minute to soften the thickened oil in the meibomian glands and dilate the opening of the glands. The oil is crucial to tear stability, improving the surface tension of the tears.
- Firm pressure applied to the closed eyelid margins through the flannel, wiping side to side to express the oil and scrub or lift adherent debris (mixture of dead skin cells and secretions) from the lashes.

In addition, lubricate the eye with artificial tear drops and treat infections when present and recommend a diet rich in Omega 3, 6 and 9.

Oral lymecycline, doxycycline or minocycline for several months.

Meibomian gland dysfunction (MGD)

Thick oily meibomian secretion causing stingy sore eyes and red thickened eyelids. Poor aqueous tear film results. Often associated with rosacea (Figure 32.4). Management is as for blepharitis, adding antibiotic for rosacea.

Upper eyelid entropion (Figure 32.5)

Mild upper eyelid entropion from chronic staphylococcal lid margin disease.

Symptoms: foreign-body lash sensation and dry, gritty eyes.

Signs: trichiasis and punctate epithelial corneal stain.

Management

- Epilation, electrolysis and cryotherapy trichiasis, medical topical lubricants and anterior lamella reposition.

Pterygium

See Figure 32.6 and also Chapter 14.

Dry eyes

Idiopathic dry eyes

Symptoms: gritty, sandy, burning dry eyes with reflex tear flooding.

Signs: poor tear film, interpalpebral punctuate epithelial staining and poor wetting on litmus paper (Schirmer's test).

Management: Vigorously treating blepharitis and meibomian gland dysfunction, use of artificial tears without preservatives and carbomeric gels, and surgical punctal occlusion with punctual plugs or punctual cautery.

Sjögren's syndrome

This exocrine gland hypofunction affects the lacrimal, salivary glands and the gastrointestinal tract. It predominantly affects women (90% cases), and the age of onset is from 35 to 55 years. Primary Sjögren's syndrome is idiopathic (approximately 50%). Secondary causes include rheumatoid arthritis, lupus or scleroderma. Symptoms are severe fatigue; dry eyes, nose and throat; dental caries and digestive problems. Vision can be impaired from epithelial damage and subsequent conjunctival and corneal scarring.

Other causes of dry eye

- Stevens–Johnson syndrome
- ocular cicatricial pemphigoid (Figure 32.8)
- lacrimal gland trauma (surgical excision or ductile destruction) and chemical, radiotherapy and thermal injury
- fibromyalgia and chronic fatigue syndrome.

Superior limbic keratitis (SLK)

The typical patient with superior limbic keratoconjunctivitis (SLK) (Figure 32.7) is female, aged 20–60 years with chronic symptoms of bilateral red and irritable eyes. It may be asymmetrical. After episodes of exacerbation and remission it usually resolves. The patient may also have abnormal thyroid function.

Management

- SLK has been treated with silver nitrate or thermal cauterisation of the superior bulbar conjunctiva, pressure patching, and large diameter bandage contact lenses (BCL), topical trans-retinoic acid 0.1%, and recession or resection of the superior bulbar conjunctiva.

• Over 50% of patients with SLK are said to have keratoconjunctivitis sicca (severe dry eye). Punctual plugs have also been used to treat SLK.

Ocular cicatricial pemphigoid (OCP) (Figure 32.8)

Severe and rare conjunctival disease which has an insidious onset with redness, grittiness and photophobia (early stages). Later, there is cicatricial entropion, severe dry eye, corneal scarring opacification and blindness. There is conjunctival fornix loss with symblepharon and reduction of eye movements. Other mucous membranes may be involved (e.g. the mouth and nasal mucosa). Treatment is with systemic immunosuppression (e.g. dapsone).

Allergic eye disease
Hayfever
This is seasonal allergic conjunctivitis, from type 1 immediate immune response with histamine release to allergens such as pollen.
Symptoms: bilateral, itchy, watery eyes with lid swelling and sometimes mucous discharge. Rhinorrhoea and sneezing. Worse in young people with atopy.
Management: topical mast cell stabilizer (e.g. sodium chromoglycate or lodoxamide).

Perennial allergic conjunctivitis
This is triggered by allergens such as house dust mites, moulds, pollens, food preservatives and animal dander. It is bilateral, with episodic symptoms. Management is the same as for hayfever, plus oral and topical antihistamine when severe.

Vernal keratoconjunctivitis sicca (VKC)
This is a young person's disease (7–11 years). Signs include characteristic upper tarsal conjunctival cobblestones (see Chapter 25), which may induce ptosis. There are often perilimbal giant papillae, known as limbal vernal. Management is as for hayfever, plus topical steroids when severe.

Acute allergic conjunctivitis
Sudden, unilateral, itchy lid swelling and marked conjunctival chemosis. Signs are worse than symptoms. Triggered by plant allergens. Resolves spontaneously without treatment within 24–36h.

KEY POINTS

- Blepharitis is a common cause of red-rimmed, itchy eyes.
- Use topical lubricant drops (hypromellose) for dry eyes.
- Excise pterygium only if encroaching onto the cornea and visual axis.

---

33 Common conditions affecting the cornea

Figure 33.1 Anatomy of the cornea

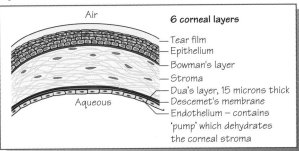

Air

6 corneal layers

- Tear film
- Epithelium
- Bowman's layer
- Stroma
- Dua's layer, 15 microns thick
- Descemet's membrane
- Endothelium – contains 'pump' which dehydrates the corneal stroma

Aqueous

Figure 33.2 Marginal keratitis

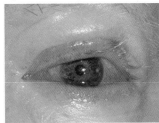

Figure 33.3 (a) Hypopyon ulcer and (b) severe bacterial keratitis with hypopyon

(a)
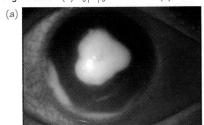

(b)
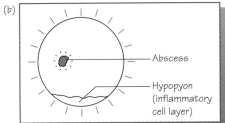

- Abscess
- Hypopyon (inflammatory cell layer)

Figure 33.4 Wessely's ring (acanthamoeba)

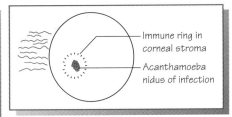

- Immune ring in corneal stroma
- Acanthamoeba nidus of infection

Figure 33.5 (a) Dendritic keratitis (herpes simplex ketatitis) and (b) corneal staining with fluorescein

(a)
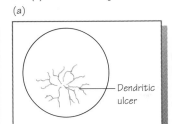

- Dendritic ulcer

(b)
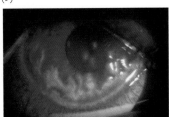

Figure 33.6 Herpes zoster ophthalmicus (HZO). (a) The area of the face affected, supplied by the first division (Vi) of the trigeminal nerve, (b) the early vesicular phase

(a)
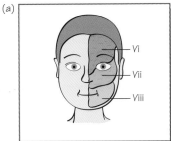

- Vi
- Vii
- Viii

Vesicles are strictly dermatomal however the swelling may spread to the other half of the face

(b)
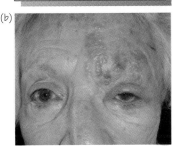

Figure 33.7 Diagram outline of a normal cornea and a keratoconic cornea, (b) Hydrops in keratocous – acute central corneal swelling and reduced vision

(a)
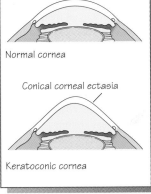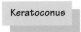

Normal cornea

Conical corneal ectasia

Keratoconic cornea

(b)
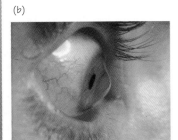

Figure 33.8 Conjunctival-corneal intraepithelial neoplasia (CCIN)

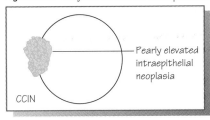

- Pearly elevated intraepithelial neoplasia

CCIN

Ophthalmology at a Glance, Second Edition. Jane Olver, Lorraine Cassidy, Gurjeet Jutley, and Laura Crawley. © 2014 Jane Olver, Lorraine Cassidy, Gurjeet Jutley and Laura Crawley. Published 2014 by John Wiley & Sons, Ltd. Companion Website: www.ataglanceseries.com/ophthal

The cornea is the window of the eye. It must be clear and healthy to function well. It requires protection by the eyelids, a healthy tear film as well as a healthy endothelial pump to keep it transparent. It is highly sensitive.

Aims

- Outline the basic anatomy of the cornea.
- Know the signs and symptoms of corneal disease.
- Describe common disease processes involving the cornea.

Exciting discovery in 2013 in the world of cornea surgery

A research group led by Professor Harminder Singh Dua has published evidence of the existence of a sixth layer of the cornea. Donor human globes had big bubbles of air injected at the layer of deep stroma. This is one of the steps in deep anterior lamellar corneal surgery, preferred method to treat anterior cornea pathology. Descemet's membrane (DM) was then removed surgically, and they noted the air dissipated in some bubbles but not others, suggesting that this bubble had been trapped between the DM and the newly described 'Dua's' layer.

Electron microscopy images revealed a fifteen 15μm microns thick collagen layer between the corneal stroma and Descemet's membrane. The composition is of 5 to 8 lamellae of type-1 collagen bundles. Dua's layer is extremely strong, capable of withstanding 200kPa of pressure.

Corneal clarity

The cornea is clear due to its highly organized structure of collagen fibres. It is free of blood vessels and allows the passage of light in an organized way so that a clear image is focused on the retina (Figure 33.1). The corneal layers all contribute to its function. The deepest endothelial cells actively pump fluid out from the stroma.

Disturbance of the eyelids, conjunctiva or tear film may lead to corneal problems, including ulceration. If corneal ulceration is severe, scarring with vascularization may lead to reduced vision and, in rare cases, to corneal perforation requiring surgical management. Corneal anaesthesia (fifth cranial nerve palsy) predisposes one to severe keratitis.

Corneal disease

Keratitis (Figures 33.2 and 33.3)

General term used to denote inflammation of the cornea from infection and inflammation.

Symptoms: pain and photosensitivity which may be absent in herpetic disease due to corneal hypoaesthesia, reduced visual acuity and/or discharge.

Signs: reduced visual acuity and circumcorneal injection—a red, inflamed eye, the presence of staining on fluorescein drop instillation, visible corneal infiltrate with or without anterior chamber hypopyon and blepharospasm.

Marginal keratitis (Figure 33.2)

This peripheral cornea ulcer is an immune reaction to chronic staphylococal lid margin disease.

Infections

Bacterial keratitis

Secondary to minor trauma (corneal abrasion or contact lens wear). *Treat as an emergency* as severe infections can lead to corneal perforation, endophthalmitis and loss of vision.

Often due to *Pseudomonas* in contact lens–related keratitis which causes rapid corneal opacification and melt in less than 24h (Figure 33.3). Rapidly identify the infective agent by C&S and treat with intensive topical antibiotics.

Acanthamoeba keratitis

Acanthamoeba is characterised by pain and causes prolonged corneal infection. It is associated with poor contact lens hygiene, daily wear soft contact lenses and especially the use of tap water in lens cleaning.

Diagnosis may require corneal biopsy and histological assessment. Look for a corneal Wessely ring using the slit lamp (Figure 33.4).

Corneal grafting may be required for chronic infection with deep corneal stromal scarring and acanthamoeba cysts.

Viral keratitis (Figure 33.5)

Herpes simplex types 1 and 2:
- Epithelial disease—dendritic ulceration.
- Stromal disease—disciform keratitis:
  ○ Immune mediated, presenting as a disc-shaped area of corneal oedema, hence the term 'disciform'
  ○ Stromal necrosis may result in scarring with vascularization, reducing corneal sensation, clarity and vision.

Treat epithelial disease with antiviral medication (e.g. aciclovir topically and/or systemically). Use topical corticosteroids judiciously for disciform keratitis.

WARNING

► **Steroid drops.** Do *not* give steroid drops in the presence of active epithelial disease as they may cause ulceration and blindness.

Herpes zoster ophthalmicus (Figure 33.6) Affects the fifth cranial nerve with segmental skin vesicles and erythema, of the upper eyelid, but not crossing the forehead midline. There is associated headache, malaise and fever. There is variable corneal involvement with conjunctivitis, seen as multiple epithelial pseudodendrites and anterior stromal infiltration responsive to topical corticosteroids. Increased risk in immunocompromised patients (e.g. HIV). Treatment is with systemic antivirals.

Inflammation

Peripheral necrotizing keratitis

Related to an underlying systemic vasculitis (e.g. rheumatoid arthritis, systemic lupus erythematosis or Wegener's granulomatosis). Peripheral destruction of corneal tissue is secondary to an ischaemic microvasculitis in the adjacent scleral and conjunctival vessels, or mediated immunologically by blood-borne factors or matrix metalloproteinases secreted into the tears. This pathological process is exacerbated by secondary Sjögren's syndrome.

Treatment: treat the underlying disease process with systemic immunosuppression. Treat corneal perforation conservatively with tissue glue, bandage contact lenses or corneal grafting.

Hereditary corneal dystrophies

Occurs in any level in the cornea: epithelial, stromal and endothelial. When severe, corneal grafting may be required to restore vision, although dystrophic changes often recur in the grafts.

Fingerprint and map-dot corneal epithelial dystrophies cause acute painful recurrent corneal erosions, particularly on waking. Other dystrophies include lattice dystrophy, with deposition of amyloid in the corneal stroma, and inherited disorders of corneal metabolism (e.g. granular and macular dystrophy).

Fuchs' endothelial dystrophy results in corneal clouding because of endothelial pump failure. The painful bullous keratopathy is treated with a bandage contact lens and eventual keratoplasty.

Keratoconus (Figure 33.7)

Common hereditary corneal dystrophy that is associated with Down's syndrome, disorders of collagen metabolism or atopic eye disease or is idiopathic. Keratoconic patients require special-fit contact lenses and, if needed, corneal grafting (Table 33.1). (See Chapters 34 and 35).

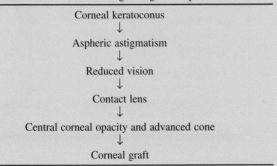

Table 33.1 Management of keratoconus: the aim is to treat with a contact lens and to avoid corneal grafting where possible

Corneal keratoconus
↓
Aspheric astigmatism
↓
Reduced vision
↓
Contact lens
↓
Central corneal opacity and advanced cone
↓
Corneal graft

Management options

- Contact lenses
- Collagen cross-linking; this recent development in the management of keratoconus is to slow disease progression. The corneal epithelium is debrided and riboflavin drops are applied, followed by ultraviolet A exposure 370 nm for 30 min to strengthen the corneal stroma by creating new collagen cross-links which helps slow deformation of the cornea.
- Intracorneal ring segments: implants made of PMMA which are placed in the corneal mid-stroma to flatten it and change the shape of the cone to reduce the astigmatism and make it less irregular. The channels to place the implants can be cut manually or by using a femtosecond laser. Typically, two arc-shaped implants are used for early keratoconus with a clear central cornea.
- Corneal graft: full-thickness graft, known as a penetrating keratoplasty (PK), or a lamellar or layered graft, known as a deep anterior lamellar keratoplasty (DALK).

Corneal neoplasia (Figure 33.8)

Conjunctival-corneal intraepithelial neoplasia (CCIN) and squamous carcinoma are important rare conditions that are more common in fairer-skinned individuals in hotter climes and in immunocompromised patients with HIV. Treatment: surgical excision or local destructive procedures.

KEY POINTS

- The healthy cornea is avascular and transparent due to the endothelial pump.
- Topical steroids may worsen dendritic keratitis and should not be used.
- Bacterial keratitis in a contact lens wearer is an emergency.

34 Medical uses of contact lenses

Figure 34.1 Keratoconus. (a) Keratoconic cornea, (b) keratoglobus and (c) corneal topography scan showing shape of a keratoconic cornea

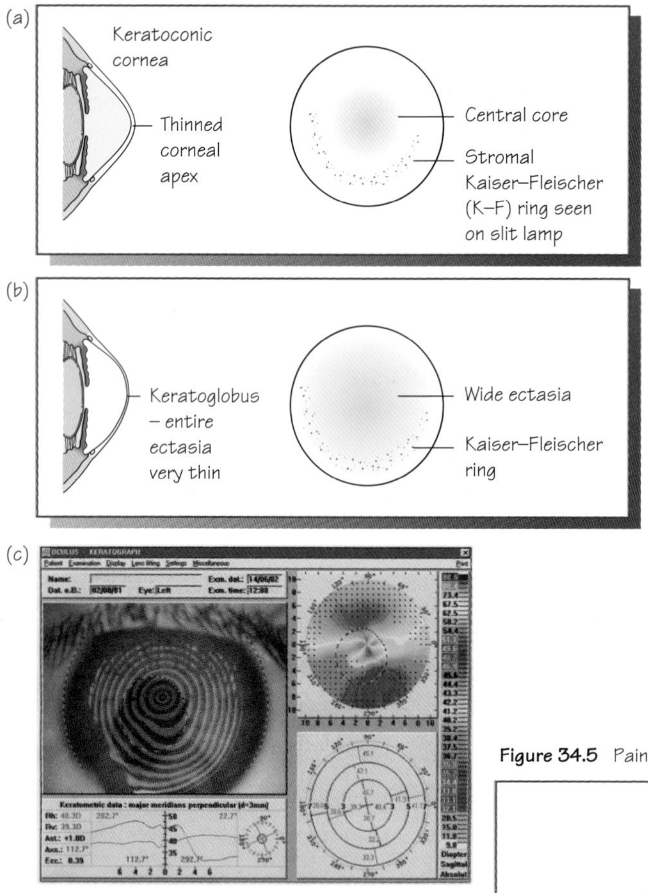
(a)
Keratoconic cornea
Thinned corneal apex
Central core
Stromal Kaiser–Fleischer (K–F) ring seen on slit lamp
(b)
Keratoglobus – entire ectasia very thin
Wide ectasia
Kaiser–Fleischer ring
(c)

Figure 34.4 Small hypopyon ulcer

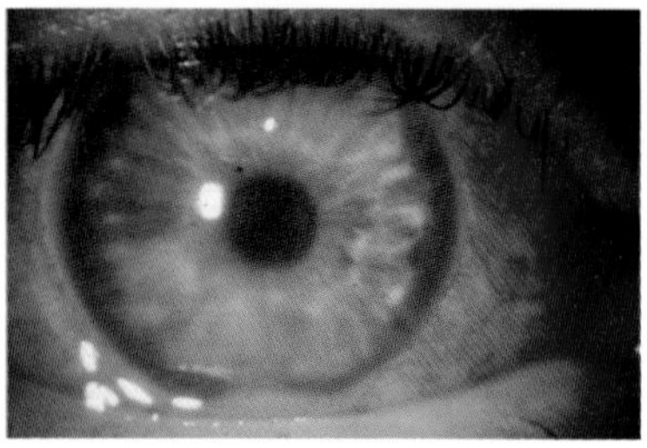

Figure 34.2 Bullous keratopathy

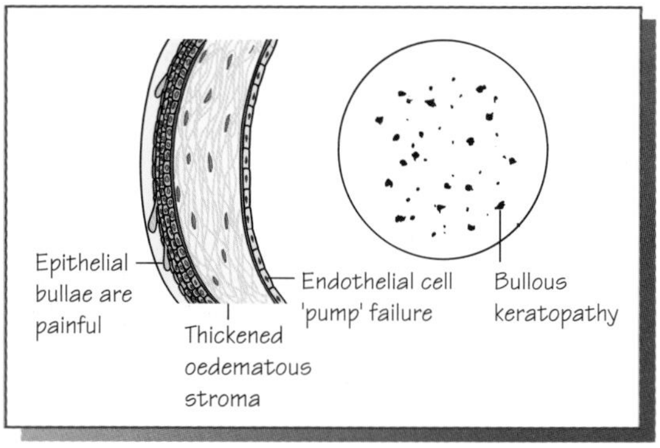
Epithelial bullae are painful
Thickened oedematous stroma
Endothelial cell 'pump' failure
Bullous keratopathy

Figure 34.3 Tight lens syndrome

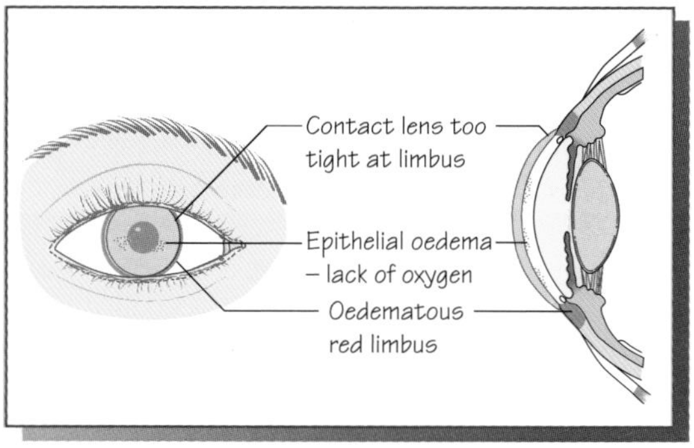
Contact lens too tight at limbus
Epithelial oedema – lack of oxygen
Oedematous red limbus

Figure 34.5 Painted contact lens

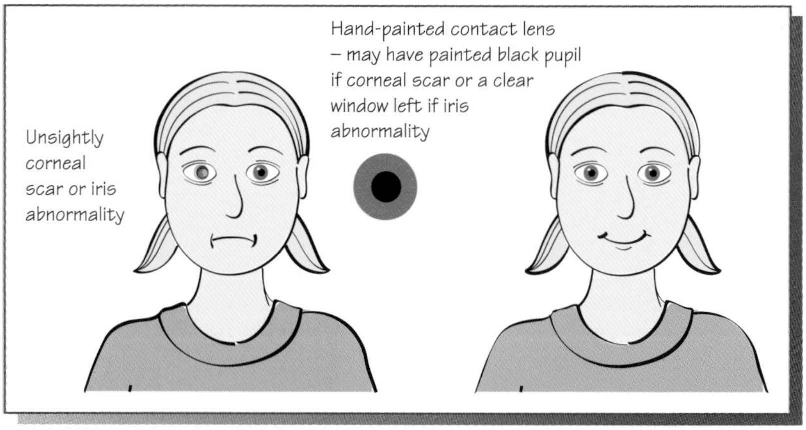
Unsightly corneal scar or iris abnormality
Hand-painted contact lens – may have painted black pupil if corneal scar or a clear window left if iris abnormality

Contact lens wear is common in the general population to correct refractive errors. They are also used as a bandage on a painful cornea and as a cosmetic prop. Unfortunately, contact lens wear can be associated with corneal morbidity.

Aims

- Medical indications for contact lenses (CL).
- Complications of contact lens wear.

Contact lenses are an excellent alternative to glasses. They are also widely used therapeutically in corneal disease. They are fitted for each patient based on the steepness and diameter of the cornea. The types of lenses (hard, gas permeable hard etc.) and materials used are summarized in Chapter 9.

Keratoconus (Figure 34.1)

In keratoconus, gas-permeable hard CL are used. Some soft CL are suitable, too, in the early stages. Once the corneal curvature is very 'steep', or the cornea is very thin, corneal graft becomes necessary (see Chapter 35).

Therapeutic bandage contact lenses

These are soft contact lenses with several functions.

Ophthalmology at a Glance, Second Edition. Jane Olver, Lorraine Cassidy, Gurjeet Jutley, and Laura Crawley. © 2014 Jane Olver, Lorraine Cassidy, Gurjeet Jutley and Laura Crawley. Published 2014 by John Wiley & Sons, Ltd. Companion Website: www.ataglanceseries.com/ophthal

Protection of normal epithelium
- Trichiasis—to prevent lashes from rubbing the cornea.
- Lid margin deformation (e.g. lower lid entropion with lashes touching the cornea, as temporary relief until surgery can be performed)
- Protection of corneal graft epithelium.
- Dry eye (e.g. pemphigoid and Stevens–Johnson syndrome).
- Exposure keratitis—following seventh cranial nerve palsy.
- To protect the cornea if there are sutures on the lid margin or under the eyelid, abrading the cornea. Use until sutures dissolve or can be removed.

Healing abnormal epithelium
- Corneal epithelial dystrophy (e.g. Cogan's microcystic epithelial dystrophy, Meesman's dystrophy, Reis–Buckler's dystrophy and map-dot or fingerpoint dystrophy).
- Chronic corneal ulcers—due to herpes simplex or vernal keratoconjunctivitis.
- Abrasions and erosions.
- Filamentary keratitis—also rapid relief of the discomfort caused by the corneal filaments.
- Chemical, thermal and irradiation burns—high high-water-content CL may be useful to restore normal epithelialization.

Moulding and splinting
- Post-keratoplasty (corneal grafting)—to flatten and reposition the graft when lifting or displacement of graft occurs.
- Wound leaks—small corneal perforations need tight fitting; post-trabeculectomy bleb leaks need large lenses to cover the leak.

Pain relief
- Bullous keratopathy—CL help to alleviate pain by covering exposed nerve endings (Figure 34.2).
- Postrefractive surgery—photorefractive keratectomy (PRK) and laser-assisted sub-epithelial keratectomy (LASEK) for pain relief and wound healing. See Chapter 35.

Complications of contact lenses
Corneal physiology
The constant metabolic activity in the cornea maintains transparency, temperature, cell reproduction and the transport of tissue materials. The main nutrients are glucose, amino acids (from the aqueous humour) and oxygen (from the tear film by diffusion when the eye is open, and from the tarsal conjunctiva when the eyelids are closed). Without oxygen, there is hypoxia or anoxia.

Hypoxia and anoxia
There are virtually no lenses available that fully meet the oxygen requirements of the cornea, and there is no CL as physiological or oxygen permeable as having no CL on the eye.

One of the first important effects of **hypoxia** (which the patient is unaware of) is a drop in corneal sensitivity. **Anoxia** causes corneal swelling, especially of the epithelium. If there is not enough oxygen available to convert glucose, by the means of glycolysis, into energy, the waste product (lactic acid) is allowed to diffuse and build up in the stroma. Sufficient osmotic pressure is created to allow water to be drawn into the stroma faster than the endothelial pump can remove it, so eventually corneal epithelial and stromal swelling occurs.

Lack of oxygen results in acute epithelial necrosis, microcystic epitheliopathy, epithelial and stromal oedema and corneal neovascularization.

Anatomical effects
Result in the following: tight lens syndrome (Figure 34.3), corneal abrasions (foreign bodies), three and nine o'clock staining (drying of corneal surface and abnormal blink), inferior corneal stain (incomplete blinking), dimple veil (static air bubble under lens) and over-wearing syndrome (mechanical and metabolic factors).

Biological activity
The presence of a CL acting as a biological active surface can cause:
- Toxic keratopathy (proteolytic enzyme—the chemical preservative in lens-cleaning solutions).
- Thiomersal keratopathy (the preservative in CL solutions or instilled eye drops acts as a hapten, causing a delayed hypersensitivity response)
- Giant papillary conjunctivitis (multifactorial aetiology—immune response to antigenic proteins on lenses and mechanical effects of lens edge) causes red sticky eye.
- Sterile corneal infiltrate—inflammatory response in the absence of an infecting organism, hypersensitivity to disinfectants and bacterial products as well as lens fit are aetiological factors.

Microbial keratitis
Caused by a complex interaction of various factors and increased ocular susceptibility and exposure to pathogens, and it is associated with *Pseudomonas*, *Staphylococcus* and *Acanthamoeba* (ubiquitous free-living protozoan). Hypopyon ulcer many occur. Even a small hypopyon ulcer can rapidly progress (Figure 34.4).

Guidelines for managing microbial conjunctivitis
Emergencies are a routine occurrence in CL practice.

> **WARNING**
>
> ▶ In a contact lens wearer, corneal and conjunctival complications are due to contact lens wear until proved otherwise.

- *Leave the lens out*—inflammatory symptoms of lens-related disease respond within a few days of ceasing lens wear.
- *Exclude microbial keratitis.*
- *Do not treat a red eye with steroids when there is a corneal ulcer.*

Advice for patients
Maintain a high standard of CL hygiene. Lenses should be cleaned and disinfected each time they are removed. Avoid overnight wear. Have back-up spectacles. Leave lenses out when adverse symptoms or a red eye develops.

Feel good—look good—see good: if these criteria are not met, the patient should seek help.

Cosmetic contact lenses
Used to hide a corneal scar or aniridia or to disguise iris abnormality (Figure 34.5). Can have a visual pupil through which the wearer can see, or it can be occlusive.

These are becoming increasingly popular, often with larger diameter coloured lenses to make the eyes look bigger cosmetically.

> **KEY POINTS**
>
> - Use bandage CL for corneal protection and to aid healing, splinting and pain relief.
> - Anoxia causes corneal swelling, cloudiness and pain.
> - Beware bacterial contact lens complications!

Figure 35.1 (a) Normal corneal limbal anatomy and (b) pterygium surgery

(a)

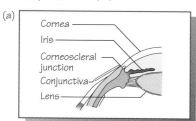

- Cornea
- Iris
- Corneoscleral junction
- Conjunctiva
- Lens

(b)

Pterygium

- Invasive pterygium
- Fibrovascular growth

Pterygium surgery

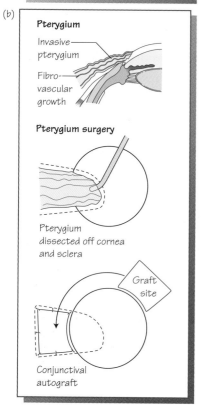

Pterygium dissected off cornea and sclera

Graft site

Conjunctival autograft

Figure 35.2 Penetrating keratoplasty. A full-thickness corneal graft in an eye that had a central corneal scar

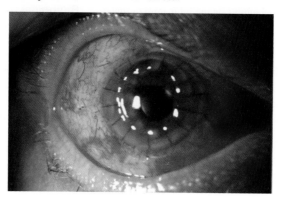

Figure 35.3 Laser refractive surgery

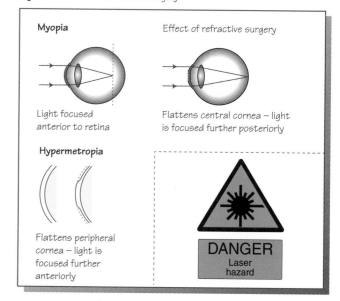

Myopia — Effect of refractive surgery

Light focused anterior to retina

Flattens central cornea – light is focused further posteriorly

Hypermetropia

Flattens peripheral cornea – light is focused further anteriorly

DANGER Laser hazard

Figure 35.4 LASer in situ keratomileusis (LASIK)

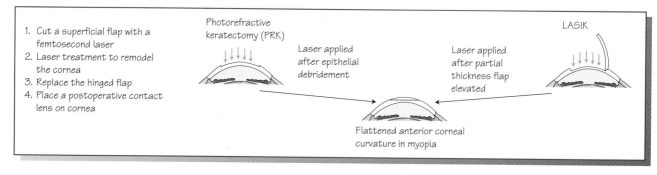

1. Cut a superficial flap with a femtosecond laser
2. Laser treatment to remodel the cornea
3. Replace the hinged flap
4. Place a postoperative contact lens on cornea

Photorefractive keratectomy (PRK)

Laser applied after epithelial debridement

LASIK

Laser applied after partial thickness flap elevated

Flattened anterior corneal curvature in myopia

Ophthalmology at a Glance, Second Edition. Jane Olver, Lorraine Cassidy, Gurjeet Jutley, and Laura Crawley. © 2014 Jane Olver, Lorraine Cassidy, Gurjeet Jutley and Laura Crawley. Published 2014 by John Wiley & Sons, Ltd. Companion Website: www.ataglanceseries.com/ophthal

This is a very exciting area of ophthalmology. With increasing numbers of people having laser refractive surgery, they have to understand the consequences of this.

Aims
- Surgical management of keratoconus.
- Principles of corneal surgery.
- Know about current laser refractive techniques.

Cornea
The healthy cornea is clear, tough and free of blood vessels or opacification and acts as an important refractive surface. Corneal clarity is dependent on the integrity and normal functioning of all five of its cellular layers (see Chapter 33). Of particular importance is the corneal endothelium, a single cell layer of non-mitotic cells that maintains the cornea in a state of partial 'dehydration' and hence transparency through the use of cellular metabolic 'pumps'. When that pump fails, the stroma swells and becomes hazy, for example in bullous keratopathy (see Chapter 34) requiring a bandage contact lens (CL) or surgery (penetrating or lamellar).

Keratitis causing corneal scarring can require PK. In order for the graft to take, the host cornea should not have many blood vessels, which could contribute to corneal graft rejection, and it should have near or near-normal sensation. A partial-thickness corneal graft is a lamellar keratoplasty.

Corneal diseases
Keratoconus
Keratoconus is the most common primary ectasia of the cornea. It is characterized by progressive thinning of the cornea, which takes on a cone formation and leads to irregular myopic astigmatism. It is a chronic progressive dystrophy that commonly starts in the second decade of life. This conical misshaping leads to astigmatism, which is variable or 'irregular' across the surface of the cornea. It is important to remember that most refraction of light occurs at the air–cornea interface rather than at the lens inside the eye, so significant changes to the cornea have a major impact on vision. Normal or 'regular' astigmatism can be corrected by glasses, but irregular astigmatism cannot. Contact lenses are usually required to make the air–cornea interface more spherical to allow the appropriate bending of the light and focusing of the eye. Early stages of the disease are usually asymptomatic and may be picked up on corneal topography, a scan which maps the corneal contours. This may be found in patients seeking corneal refractive surgery where a preoperative corneal topography scan is mandatory. Patients with keratoconus, even if it is asymptomatic, should not have LASIK as this treatment thins the cornea further and makes the keratoconus worse.

Signs
- Usually bilateral but asymmetrical.
- Vogt striae: fine vertical lines in the centre of the cornea.
- Fleischer ring: epithelial deposits of iron around the base of the cone.
- 'Oil droplet' reflex on direct ophthalmoscopy.
- 'Scissors' reflex on retinoscopy.
- Munson sign: bulging of the lower eyelid on downgaze. This is usually seen only in advanced disease, where the cone shape of the cornea pushes against the lower lid when the eye moves into downgaze.
- Stromal scarring: this is usually seen when there has been a rupture of Descemet's membrane, the membrane just outside the endothelial

layer of the cornea. When this occurs, the cornea becomes painful and oedematous as the pump function of the endothelial cells is disrupted.

Associations
- Down syndrome
- Ehlers–Danlos syndrome
- Marfan's syndrome
- osteogenesis imperfecta
- general atopy and vernal keratoconjunctivitis.

Management options
- Contact lenses.
- Collagen crosslinking; this technique uses riboflavin drops on the eye, which is then exposed to ultraviolet A light. It can stabilize or prevent progression of early forms of the condition.
- Corneal ring segment implants (e.g. Intacs®). These implants are placed into pre-cut tunnels within the stroma of the cornea to alter its shape.
- Corneal graft. This may be a full-thickness graft known as PK, or a lamellar or layered graft known as a deep anterior lamellar keratoplasty (DALK).

Pterygium (Figure 25.1b)
Microscopic lamella excision (Figure 25.1c) is needed if it encroaches on the visual axis (see Chapter 14) and corneal neoplasia (see Chapter 31).

Corneal surgery
Corneal grafting
From human donor material. Donor eyes are stored in eye banks (e.g. in London, Bristol, Manchester and Dublin). Donors are screened as all human tissue transplant material is.
- PK (Figure 35.2): a full-thickness transplant of all five layers of the cornea. This can be used for corneal dystrophies or perforations.
- DALK: replacing the anterior two-thirds of the cornea only. The recipient retains his or her own corneal endothelium, Descemet's layer and some very deep stroma. This transplant is suitable for conditions that affect the anterior portion of the cornea only (e.g. keratoconus or a corneal scar following infection). The advantages of this graft include less rejection risk and the absence of a full-thickness wound in the cornea, which can separate if the grafted eye is subjected to trauma postoperatively. The main disadvantage is that there will always be an interface between the donor anterior portion of the cornea and the recipient's retained posterior portion of the cornea, and this can impact vision. It is more difficult to perform than PK.
- Endothelial keratoplasty (Descemet's stripping endothelial keratoplasty (DSEK) or Descemet's stripping automated endothelial keratoplasty (DSAEK)): this graft is used in patients whose endothelial layer of pumps has failed and who have consequent corneal cloudiness. Only the inner layer of the cornea is transplanted.

Refractive surgery (Figure 35.3)
Surgery and/or laser is used to reshape the main refractive surface of the eye (the anterior corneal surface), and to bring light rays in focus on the retina without the need for glasses or contact lenses.

The main indication is **myopia**.

There are three methods of laser, in all of which the **excimer laser** is used to correct myopia, hypermetropia and astigmatism under local anaesthesia.

In myopia, the corneal surface is flattened so that the image focuses onto the retina. The effect in hypermetropia is not always stable.

Photorefractive keratectomy (PRK)
Excimer laser ablation reshapes the anterior corneal surface after manual debridement of the epithelium.
- Suitable for low refractive errors (−1 to −6 D).
- Disappointing for hypermetropia.
- Bandage contact lenses as eye painful for 48 h.
- Variable slow healing and remodelling over months.
- Quality of vision—temporary haze common after treatment.
- Regression can occur in higher degrees of myopia (>−10D).
- Recurrent erosions are a complication.

Laser surgery
Laser-assisted intrastromal in situ keratomileusis (LASIK) (Figure 35.4) A partial-thickness corneal-hinged epithelial 'cap' is raised, and the excimer laser ablation is applied to stromal tissue below this, after which the 'cap' is replaced.
- Suitable for higher degrees of myopia with less risk of regression (up to −10D).
- Disappointing for hypermetropia.
- No haze.
- Best visual acuity achieved more rapidly than with PRK.
- Dry eye for a few months.

Laser epithelium keratomileusis (LASEK) This can be used for low myopia and hypermetropia and in patients who are unsuitable for LASIK. The epithelium is treated with alcohol to loosen it. It is preserved with the intention of replacing it when the stroma has been ablated with the excimer laser.

Femtosecond-assisted LASIK This differs from LASIK in that the flap is 'cut' using a laser rather than a blade known as a micro-keratome. The proposed advantages include more accurate thickness of the flap and lower probability of incomplete flap or button-hole of the flap.

Blended vision
Laser blended vision, is a sophisticated laser eye treatment which rectifies short-sightedness (myopia) in one eye and long-sightedness (hyperopia) in the other eye. Primarily the treatment is for presbyopia, the progressive loss of the ability to focus on nearby objects around aged 45–50 years.

Blended vision can be achieved through laser eye surgery such as LASIK, PRK or LASEK, by correcting the dominant eye and the shape of the cornea, modifying it for reading vision and still maintaining good distance vision. In other words, one eye is focused for distance and the other eye is focused for near vision. The eyes are effectively working together to allow good vision at near, intermediate and far, without needing glasses. The effects of blended vision treatment can last between 5 to 10 years.

Who can have laser refractive surgery?
- Patients should be >21 years old, have a stable refraction, not be pregnant and have no keratoconus, cataract or glaucoma.
- They should not be on systemic steroids.
- Patients should have realistic expectations and have been warned of potential side effects of haze, night-time glare, ghosting images, starburst around lights, dry eye and risk of macular haemorrhage.
- It is also essential that patients are warned that intraocular pressure and A-scan and biometry measurements cannot be made accurately after refractive surgery.

WARNING

▶ Corneal refractive surgery can have serious, potentially sight-threatening complications as with any ocular surgery.
▶ Lasered donor eyes are not accepted for corneal grafting.
▶ Refractive surgery effects may regress with time.
▶ Patients who have laser refractive surgery for myopia will require glasses to correct their presbyopia when older than 45–50 years.

KEY POINTS

- A healthy corneal endothelium is essential for corneal clarity.
- Corneal grafting is successful, particularly in keratoconus patients.
- The main indication for laser refractive surgery is myopia.

36 Cataract assessment

Anatomy

The crystalline **lens** is composed of an inner nucleus (of older inactive cells) and an outer cortex, with the whole structure being encapsulated.
The **epithelium** is active metabolically, it synthesizes protein for **lens fibres**, transports amino acids and maintains a cation pump to keep the lens clear. At the equator of the lens, epithelial cells differentiate into lens fibres, which lose their organelles and ability for aerobic metabolism.
Zonule filaments suspend the lens **ciliary processes** to the **ciliary muscle**. When the muscle contracts the filaments relax allowing the lens to become more convex with a shorter focal length for reading

Figure 36.1 (a) Diagram of normal anterior segment, (b) close up of normal lens cross-section and (c) lens with cataract

(a)

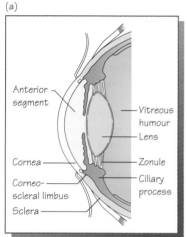
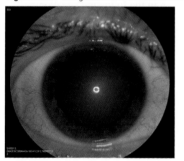

(b)

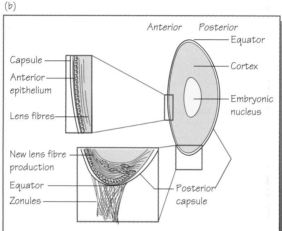
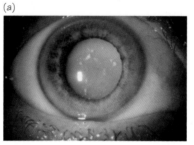

(c)

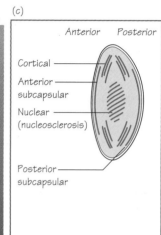
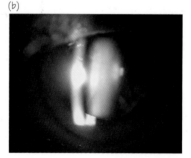

Figure 36.2 Congenital blue dot cataract

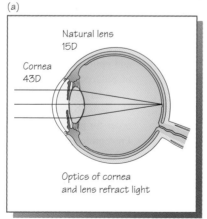

Figure 36.3 (a, b) Slit lamp view of dense cataracts

(a)

(b)

Figure 36.4 (a, b) Biometry to calculate the power of the intraocular lens

(a)

(b)

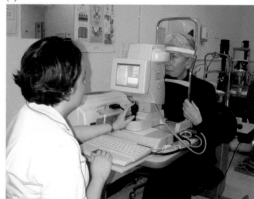

Ophthalmology at a Glance, Second Edition. Jane Olver, Lorraine Cassidy, Gurjeet Jutley, and Laura Crawley. © 2014 Jane Olver, Lorraine Cassidy, Gurjeet Jutley and Laura Crawley. Published 2014 by John Wiley & Sons, Ltd. Companion Website: www.ataglanceseries.com/ophthal

Cataract causes gradual loss of vision in a white eye in older persons. Learn to assess if a patient has a cataract using a direct ophthalmoscope.

Aims
• Appreciate the gross anatomy of the crystalline lens.
• Understand there are important causes that can accelerate the formation of cataracts.
• Know the factors considered before surgery.

The term 'cataract' is derived from the Latin word for waterfall, 'cataracta', as it is believed that the appearance of pathological lens opacities is akin to that of the magnificent waterfalls seen in nature. Other than refractive error, cataract is the most common cause of visual morbidity in adults worldwide. We are fortunate in the United Kingdom, where treatment can be given quickly and efficiently once symptoms are too troublesome for patients. Currently, cataract surgery is the most commonly performed ophthalmic surgical procedure in the United Kingdom.

Definition

Cataract: Opacity of the lens of the eye, which occurs when fluid gathers between the lens fibres. The refractive index alters and causes light scatter with resultant blurred vision. Acquired lens changes occur in 95% of people over the age of 65; however, not all of these people will require cataract surgery.

Anatomy (Figure 36.1)
• Think of the human lens as a peanut M&M held in position at the sides by the zonules extending from the ciliary body. The outer crystal coating is analogous to the lens capsule, the chocolate is equivalent to the lens cortex and the peanut is the nucleus!
• Surgically, we delicately tear a hole in the front part of the lens capsule in order to access the deeper parts of the lens: the idea is to leave the remaining lens capsule in place as a bag to support the implanted plastic intraocular lens (IOL).
• Cataracts are classified depending on the part of the lens that's opacified:
  ○ cortical
  ○ posterior subcapsular
  ○ nuclear sclerotic.

Causes of cataract
• Old age (commonest).
• Associated with other ocular and systemic diseases.
• Associated with systemic medication (steroids and phenothiazines), discussed further on in this chapter.
• Trauma and intraocular foreign bodies.
• Ionizing radiation (X-ray and UV).
• Congenital (dominant, sporadic or part of a syndrome, abnormal galactose metabolism or hypoglycaemia).
• Associated with inherited abnormality (myotonic dystrophy, Marfan's syndrome, Lowe's syndrome, rubella and high myopia).

Risk factors
All individuals will develop a cataract if they live long enough. However, certain circumstances accelerate the development of a cataract. It is important that in any referral letter these issues are highlighted, so the surgeon can be prepared pre-operatively (e.g. previous trauma may suggest weak zonules).

• Systemic causes:
  ○ diabetes mellitus
  ○ myotonic dystrophy
  ○ Wilson's disease.
• Ocular causes:
  ○ inflammatory eye disease
  ○ previous ocular surgery.
• Trauma
• Congenital conditions:
  ○ metabolic disorders.
• Drug history:
  ○ steroids
  ○ amioderone
  ○ phenothiazines.

Natural history of cataract
Typically, the nuclear sclerotic cataracts increase the refractive power of the eye, so-called refractive myopia. Hence, initially optometrists in the community can manage cataracts by prescribing greater minus lenses. If there are no other ophthalmic morbidities, these patients do not need a referral.

At this stage, examination with the direct ophthalmoscope in General Practice or Accident & Emergency will reveal an abnormally dim red reflex. Nuclear cataract causes a central black shadow, whilst cortical cataracts cause black spoke-like shadows coming from the edge of the red reflex. These spokes are also seen in the visually insignificant, congenital opacity termed a 'blue-dot cataract' (Figure 36.2).

There will come a time when spectacles alone cannot correct the refractive error: it is at this time that patients should be referred to the eye clinic for cataract surgery. If patients delay presentation, the cataracts will become dense, mature and brunescent (Figure 36.3).

Surgery should be undertaken in the following situations:
• Symptoms of:
  ○ reduced best-corrected visual acuity (BCVA) less than 6/9
  ○ monocular diplopia
  ○ Glare in sunshine or with street or car lights (particularly with dense posterior subcapsular cataracts across the visual axis).
  ○ Clouding of vision (particularly with cortical lens opacities).
• Patients with diabetes mellitus
  ○ otherwise, retinopathy changes cannot be monitored.
• Treating phacomorphic glaucoma
  ○ A large, swollen lens can physically cause the iris to bow forward. This results in a narrowing of the irido-corneal angle and a subsequent rise in the intraocular pressure (IOP) due to poor aqueous outflow.
• Patients with poor BCVA due to other causes:
  ○ All patients undergoing surgery should have dilated fundoscopy and optical coherence tomography examinations to look for causes of reduced BCVA other than cataracts, such as macular scarring secondary to age-related macular degeneration. In this scenario, although vision cannot be improved, surgery may be considered in order for patients to have better colour contrast.
• Preventing amblyopia:
  ○ A cataract in children will cause stimulus deprivation amblyopia.

TIP
• Patients with cataracts have normal pupil reflexes if there is no other ocular or optic nerve disease.

Preparation for cataract surgery

Each member of the team needs to play an active role for surgery to be successful:

- Biometry (Figure 36.4):
  - Arguably, this is the most important part of surgery. Usually, the nursing staff perform an ultrasound measurement of the length of the eye and keratometry to measure the curvature of the cornea. This enables the surgeon to decide which strength of lens should be implanted and where on the cornea the incision should be made (see Chapter 37).
- Medical pre-assessment:
  - Warfarin should not be stopped, but the international normalized ratio (INR) should be within the therapeutic range.
  - One must know if the patient is on tamsulosin, as this causes floppy iris syndrome and makes the surgery more technically difficult. Tamsulosin is the only alpha-receptor antagonist to have this effect.
  - Confirm that general medical conditions are stable, particularly hypertension, respiratory disease and diabetes. Remember that this is elective surgery and unless a patient can lie supine for 20 minutes, surgery should be reconsidered.
- Informed consent:
  - The operating surgeon should inform patients of expected outcome and the complications of surgery.
  - The surgeon should take great lengths in discussing the theatre environment and procedure steps so the patient does not feel apprehensive throughout. Remember that the operation will occur whilst the patient is awake, and this can be very unnerving. So take time to explain that:
    - There will be a drape over their head, but oxygen will be supplemented underneath.
    - They will hear talking amongst the staff in order to carry out the procedure safely.
    - There will be various members of the team in the theatre, including nurses, operating department practitioners, anaesthetists, junior doctors and medical students.
    - During parts of the operation, they will hear buzzing sounds. Furthermore, they will receive constant irrigation in the eye, and sometimes this may trickle down into their ear.
    - If they wish to move or cough, to let you know in advance to enable the safe removal of instruments outside the eye before they do so.

Biometry: intraocular lens power calculation

The desired implant should produce a sharp image on the retina. Since each eye has a different corneal curvature and axial length, the implant size has to be measured preoperatively in each patient. The optics of the eye are such that light is refracted by the cornea (effective power of 43D) and by the natural lens (effective power 15D); both of these together give the total power of the focusing components of the eye. A special equation is used to calculate the intraocular lens power, which is usually in the range of 19–22D, with some very shortsighted eyes needing lower powers and longsighted eyes needing higher powers for clear-focused distance vision.

KEY POINTS

- Cataract is common; it is one of the three main causes of blindness worldwide.
- It can occur at any age and in all races.
- It is effectively treated by glasses in the early stages and by surgery when more advanced.

37 Cataract surgery

Figure 37.1 Model of eye showing anterior chamber depth

Epithelium

Endothelium

Anterior chamber depth

Corneoscleral limbus

TIP

- Most adult cataract surgery is done under topical or local anaesthesia. The patient may see bright lights and different colours, shadows of the surgeon's hands moving or complete darkness during surgery
- Phacoemulsification lens surgery with small, foldable intraocular lens implants is the gold standard. It gives rapid visual rehabilitation with a low complication rate

Figure 37.2 Intraocular lens

Capsulorhexis edge
Intraocular lens placed in bag
Anterior capsule
Iris
Ciliary body
Zonule
Posterior capsule

Anterior capsule
Capsulorhexis edge
Intraocular in capsular bag

Figure 37.3 Steps in cataract surgery. (a) Small feather blade to make the side incision (paracentesis), (b) vision blue dye is injected to stain the capsule in difficult cataracts, (c) first vertical step of the main incision, (d) main incision, (e) start of the capsulorrhexis, (f) continuation of the capsulorrhexis, (g) hydrodissection of the plane between the capsule and the cataract, (h) emulsification of the cataract, (i) dividing the lens and cracking it into segments, (j) removing the last quadrant of the divided lens, (k) removing the residual soft lens matter, (l) implanting the intraocular lens, (m) dialling the lens into the bag and (n) administration of subconjunctival antibiotic

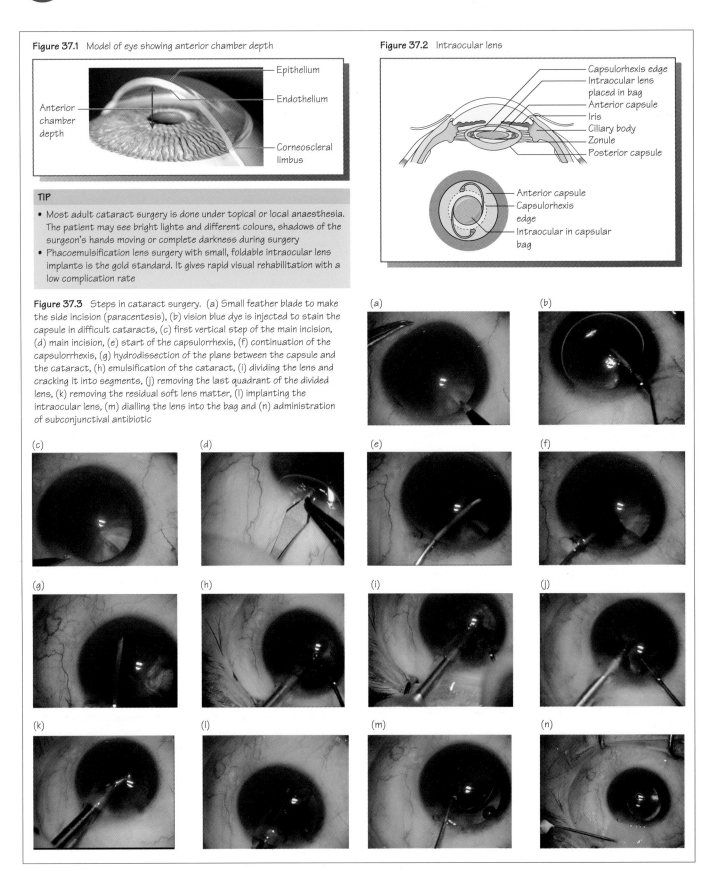

(a) (b) (c) (d) (e) (f) (g) (h) (i) (j) (k) (l) (m) (n)

Ophthalmology at a Glance, Second Edition. Jane Olver, Lorraine Cassidy, Gurjeet Jutley, and Laura Crawley. © 2014 Jane Olver, Lorraine Cassidy, Gurjeet Jutley and Laura Crawley. Published 2014 by John Wiley & Sons, Ltd. Companion Website: www.ataglanceseries.com/ophthal

Aims

- Understand the methods of anaesthesia.
- Understand the principles of cataract removal.
- Be able to explain cataract surgery to a patient.

Microsurgery in developed countries has reached a very high standard due to the developments in microsurgical instruments and intraocular lens design. There is controlled and precise removal of the lens with the assistance of an operating microscope. The majority of the lens capsule is retained to hold the implant within it. An operating microscope is needed. In order to reach the lens, a small corneal incision is made close to the limbus for the phacoemulsification (phaco) probe. It is important to appreciate the anterior chamber depth and to keep all instruments away from the corneal endothelium, in the plane of the iris (Figure 37.1).

Definitions

- Phakia: an eye with a natural lens *in situ*.
- Pseudophakia: an eye that has had a cataract removed and an artificial intraocular lens implanted (Figure 37.2).
- Aphakia: an eye that has had a cataract removed without an artificial lens inserted.

Anaesthesia for cataract surgery

Local anaesthesia

- Topical: drops of proxymethocaine; there is full kinesis of the extraocular muscles (EOM), and hence you need a compliant patient and a confident surgeon.
- Subtenons: dissect through the conjunctiva and Tenon's capsule, inferomedially. Use a blunt cannula to administer 2 ml of lidocaine within this plane.
- Peribulbar injection: a 21-gauge needle is used to distribute 5–10 ml lidocaine within the orbit. It can be administered via the skin or through the conjunctiva.
- Retrobulbar injection: direct 1–2 ml lidocaine within the muscle cone. This is now becoming less commonly used, due to the risk of retro-bulbar haemorrhage.

Sedation

Intravenous drugs may be given with local anaesthetics but are not preferred as the patient could drift off to sleep and then suddenly wake up with a jolt and move his or her head—which is undesirable in cataract surgery.

General anaesthesia

This is used for young and uncooperative patients.

Surgical technique for cataract removal

- Patients have to lie supine so a microscope with a bright light and good magnification can be positioned above them.
- The surgeon works from the side or above the head, looking down the microscope, using the red reflex from the retina to aid cataract removal.
- Operating superiorly, the surgeon has the advantage of support for his or her hands from the patients' brow. However, deeper set eyes are difficult to access because of this.
- Temporally, the surgeon has the advantage of less restriction of hand movements. Conversely, he or she lacks support for stabilization.
- The incision should be made dependent on the keratometry result of the patient. Operate on the steeper axis as the incision will flatten this axis and steepen the cornea 90° to this: this phenomenon is called 'coupling'. Both effects act to reduce the astigmatic error.

Draping

Before surgery can start, the eyelids and lashes are covered with a thin transparent plastic drape in order to keep contaminated lashes out of the surgical field. Staphylococci live in abundance on the lashes. The drape is light and also covers the face—lifted up from it as a small tent—to protect the face from irrigation fluids used in the surgery, which are collected into a small bag at the side of the head.

Small speculum

The eyelids are kept open by a combination of the drape and a small wire speculum, which does not cause the patient discomfort.

Surgery (Figure 37.3)

- Extracapsular cataract surgery is very rarely used in the United Kingdom now. The procedure involves removal of the entire nucleus as one piece; the soft cortex is aspirated, and a rigid or soft implant is inserted. The corneal wound is large and requires sutures to close, which are removed as late as 8 weeks after surgery.
- Small incision sutureless cataract surgery (SISCS) is not used in the United Kingdom but is commonly used in places like India. The surgery involves creating a long scleral tunnel and expressing the nucleus as a whole. A phaco machine is not required in this technique.
- Phacoemulsification and intraocular lenses (IOLs) comprise the technique of choice in the United Kingdom, and trainees are taught this from the ST1 level. The steps are highlighted on the diagrams, but briefly:
  ○ The main incision is made by a keratome and is about 3 mm in size (small incision).
  ○ A small needle (cystotome) is used to create a circular hole in the front part of the lenticular capsule.
  ○ A cannula is used to inject water in the plane between the lens and capsule (a process called hydrodissection).
  ○ The lens is cracked into small fragments using a sharp chopper and the main phaco probe. Techniques used commonly are divide and conquer, stop and chop and vertical chop.
  ○ Fragments are irrigated through the probe, followed by the soft lens matter adherent to the inner capsule.
  ○ A soft, foldable IOL implant can be inserted through the small incision into the remaining lens capsule (posterior chamber IOL). This incision is usually sutureless.

Implant power

The IOL power is carefully calculated to take into account the patient's postoperative visual requirements. After surgery, the lens is unable to accommodate, so the patient and surgeon decide preoperatively what type of vision the surgery should aim for. Most commonly, patients choose to be left emmetropic for distance and need glasses to read. Emphasize that whilst all efforts are made to achieve this aim, the surgeon cannot guarantee a particular result and the patient may require glasses to also refine distance vision.

Multifocal IOLs (for both near and far correction) are available but not commonly used. Toric lenses are used more readily, in order to correct astigmatism that is too great to be corrected solely by placing the primary incision along the steep axis. In practice, steepening of greater than 2 dioptres merits thought of using a toric lens.

KEY POINTS

- Microsurgery: the replacement of the natural lens with an artificial one.
- The day case procedure is performed under local anaesthesia.
- Patient needs to be able to lie still and flat for approx 20 min.
- Watch a cataract surgery at least once on your attachment.

Table 38.1 Symptoms, signs and treatment of early postoperative problems

Early postoperative problems	Symptom	Sign	Treatment
Raised intraocular pressure	Pain, deep ache, blurred vision	Hazy cornea	Ophthalmologist needs to measure pressure and treat with systemic acetazolamide 250 mg 2–4 times daily (1–2 days) and glaucoma drops
Leaking incision	Poor vision	Siedel positive with fluorescein	Ophthalmologist may need to suture the wound in the operating theatre. If the anterior chamber is deep and the ocular pressure is normal, a soft contact lens may be placed on the eye. Daily review is required
Subconjunctival haemorrhage	Red eye, no pain	Diffuse redness on the globe	Continue drops. Reinforce good technique for instilling drops
Corneal oedema	Poor vision	Hazy cornea	Ophthalmologist needs to exclude raised pressure and increase topical steroid drops
Epithelial erosion (conjunctiva or cornea)	Gritty, watering	Fluorescein staining; may have injected bulbar conjunctiva	Continue drops and reassure. Monitor carefully to exclude early infection
Conjunctivitis	Pain, redness with mucopurulent discharge	Swollen, red tarsal conjunctiva while maintaining good vision	Prescribe different antibiotic, (e.g. ofloxacin) to be used twice hourly. Frequent review to confirm no progression to endophthalmitis

Table 38.2 Symptoms, signs and treatment of sight-threatening postoperative problems that require urgent treatment by an ophthalmologist

Sight-threatening postop problems requiring urgent treatment by ophthalmologist	Symptom	Signs observed with pen torch	Slit lamp signs observed by ophthalmologist	Treatment (by ophthalmologist)
Endophthalmitis	Painful, red eye usually with a mucopurulent discharge and poor vision at day 3–5	Red eye with hazy cornea. A relative afferent pupillary defect indicates serious visual damage	Flare, cells and hypopyon in the anterior chamber	URGENT in-patient management. Intensive topical broad-spectrum antibiotics (drops). Requires aqueous and vitreous sample for microscopy, culture and sensitivity
Macular oedema (retina)	Poor vision during first 60 days after surgery	Normal anterior segment of the eye	Slit lamp fundus examination and fluorescein angiography show increased fluid in the retina around the fovea	Treated with anti-inflammatory drops (steroid and non-steroidal), steroid injection around the eye, and systemic non-steroidal anti-inflammatory (neurofen)
Opacity of posterior part of the original epithelial capsule of the natural lens (can occur between 1 month and 2 years after surgery)	Gradual deterioration of vision, as though cataract is reforming	White eye with no external abnormality. Red reflex from fundus may be obscured	Posterior capsule hazy or white. Implant is unaffected	Make a hole in the capsule using a YAG laser (clinic procedure requiring anaesthetic drops). Cornea, anterior chamber and implant are not affected by the laser

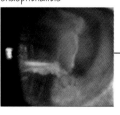

Figure 38.1 Hypopyon indicates endophthalmitis

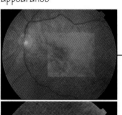

Figure 38.2 Fibrin plaque: intense postoperative inflammation in endophthalitis

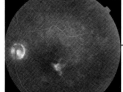

Figure 38.3 Cystoid macular oedema (CMO). (a) Typical colour fundus and (b) fluorescein angiographic appearance

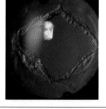

Figure 38.4 YAG capsulotomy hole made in a thickened posterior capsule

Although cataract surgery is technically highly specialized, there still can be complications which are sight threatening.

Aims
- Be aware of normal and undesirable postoperative events.
- Recognize postoperative complications from history.

Routine postoperative management
Patients are discharged as day cases and are usually given a clear shield to wear over the operated eye. Steroids and antibiotic drops are administered four times daily for 2–4 weeks after surgery. During that time, patients can read, take gentle exercise, shop, shower or bath and wash their hair carefully. Spectacles can be prescribed from 6 weeks after surgery.

Undesirable postoperative events (complications)
Watering and a foreign body sensation are common after surgery (Table 38.1).

As with any surgical complications, think about them in time order:
- Acute:
  - Endophthalmitis (Table 38.2):
    - an intraocular infection of the whole eye
    - This is the most important sight-threatening complication following surgery and requires urgent admission and treatment.
    - Its onset is usually 4–5 days after surgery. The most common organism causing endophthalmitis is coagulase-negative *Staphylococcus*, particularly *S. epidermidis*.
    - The signs and symptoms that one should look for in such patients are:
      - severe pain
      - loss of vision
      - injected conjunctiva
      - hypopyon (Figure 38.1)
      - intense inflammation and fibrin plaque formation (Figure 38.2)
      - loss of red reflex.
- Subacute:
  - Postoperative cystoid macular oedema (CMO) or Irvine–Gass syndrome (Figure 38.3 and Table 38.2);

- Classically, this occurs at 6 weeks postoperatively.
- The vision, which had hitherto been clear following surgery, suddenly drops, and the patient complains of distortion.
- Treatment involves topical steroids, non-steroidal anti-inflammatory drugs and carbonic anhydrase inhibitors (CAIs).
- Chronic (months to years following surgery):
  - Posterior capsular opacification (PCO) (Table 38.2);
    - The bag containing the lens implant (the remaining part of the capsule) over time can accumulate mucopolysaccharides. Certain intraocular lenses have a greater tendency to do this, and the risk is increased if strands of soft lens matter are left in situ during surgery.
    - Patients describe a frosted appearance of their vision and have symptoms similar to their original cataract formation (a so-called after-cataract).
    - Treatment is a simple yttrium–aluminium–garnet capsulotomy laser procedure (Figure 38.4).
  - Rhegmatogenous retinal detachment (RRD);
    - 1.5% of patients undergoing surgery develop retinal detachment. This is particularly pertinent if the posterior capsule (PC) was breached inadvertently during surgery and vitreous spilled over into the anterior chamber (a so-called PC tear).
  - Bullous keratopathy;
    - This is associated with complicated surgery.
    - The surgical field that ophthalmologists operate in is about 3 mm from the endothelial cells of the cornea to the anterior capsule of the lens. If the surgeon is not extremely careful, some of the endothelium can be scraped off during surgery.
    - The endothelium contains pumps to continually remove fluid back out to the AC.
    - If enough cells are scraped off, eventually the cornea decompensates, becomes cloudy and develops painful bullae.

KEY POINTS

- Endophthalmitis is the most serious postoperative complication.
- Advise patients to have refraction 6 weeks post-surgery.
- Be aware of the long-term complications of cataract surgery.

Figure 39.1 Anatomy: aqueous production, drainage and resistance to flow

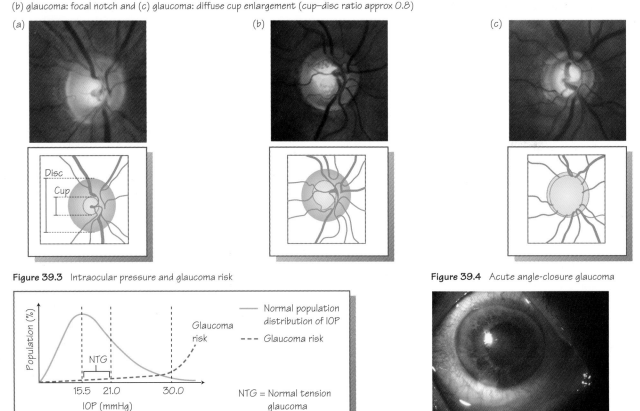

Intraocular pressure (IOP) is a balance of aqueous production and clearance. Aqueous humour is produced by the ciliary body. Aqueous flows forward over the anterior surface of the lens, through the pupil and drains through the trabecular meshwork into Schlemm's canal. The alternative uveoscleral pathway drains 10% of aqueous

Sites of blockage:
1 Ciliary block
2 Pupil block
3 Pre-trabecular – neovascular membrane or cellular debris
4 Trabecular
5 Post-trabecular – elevated episcleral venous pressure

Figure 39.2 Normal and cupped optic nerve heads in chronic primary open angle glaucoma. (a) Normal disc (cup–disc ratio approx 0.3), (b) glaucoma: focal notch and (c) glaucoma: diffuse cup enlargement (cup–disc ratio approx 0.8)

Figure 39.3 Intraocular pressure and glaucoma risk

Figure 39.4 Acute angle-closure glaucoma

Glaucoma is not just one eye condition.

Aims
- Understand the group of conditions classed as glaucoma.
- Know the symptoms and signs of acute angle-closure glaucoma to enable urgent referral for treatment of this ophthalmic emergency.

Definitions
Glaucoma affects 60 million people worldwide: 8.4 million bilaterally blind from chronic glaucoma. Commonest cause of irreversible blindness in the world, affecting 2% of people over 40 years of age and 4% of people over 70 years. Glaucoma is a multifactorial optic neuropathy with characteristic acquired loss of optic nerve fibres causing structural change in the optic nerve and functional change with loss of visual field. The intraocular pressure (Figure 39.1) may be, but is not necessarily, elevated.

Intraocular pressure (IOP): the 'normal' range of IOP is defined as 10–21 mmHg. Patients with IOP within the 'normal range' may develop glaucoma (often referred to as 'normal tension glaucoma'), and some patients with IOP above the 'normal range' do not develop optic nerve damage (ocular hypertension). Elevated IOP is still a risk factor for the development of glaucoma, and when glaucomatous damage is observed treatment is reduction of IOP regardless of the absolute presenting value.

Ophthalmology at a Glance, Second Edition. Jane Olver, Lorraine Cassidy, Gurjeet Jutley, and Laura Crawley. © 2014 Jane Olver, Lorraine Cassidy, Gurjeet Jutley and Laura Crawley. Published 2014 by John Wiley & Sons, Ltd. Companion Website: www.ataglanceseries.com/ophthal

Ocular hypertension (OHT)

Patients with raised IOP but no signs of glaucomatous optic neuropathy have OHT. It is common to find that they have thicker than average corneas. In the Ocular Hypertension Treatment study 10–20% of patients with OHT developed glaucoma, and 80% did not develop structural or functional damage.

Skills to obtain

• Use of direct ophthalmoscope to evaluate disc colour, contour and cup-to-disc ratio.

Classification

The glaucomas are a diverse group of eye conditions (at least 60 types) defined in diagnostic groups:

• primary or secondary: the presence or absence of causative factors
• open-angle or angle-closure: the anatomy of the drainage angle
• acute or chronic: speed of onset
• age of onset: congenital, juvenile or adult.

Primary open-angle glaucoma (POAG)

Commonest glaucoma in Caucasian and Afro-Caribbean populations. The exact pathogenesis is unknown; various factors are implicated, including elevated IOP and altered blood supply to the optic nerve. Genetics play a role, with nine loci in the human genome associated with glaucoma. Risk factors include elevated IOP, thin cornea, positive family history and Afro-Caribbean descent.

Symptoms

Glaucoma is asymptomatic until advanced with marked optic disc cupping (Figure 39.2) and extensive visual field loss. Central vision is preserved until a late stage.

Signs

• Usually, but not necessarily, raised IOP (Figure 39.3).
• Normal open angle on gonioscopy.
• Characteristic optic disc changes including progressive thinning of the optic disc neurosensory rim indicating loss of nerve fibres. Typically, the inferior and superior rims thin first and may give the appearance of a notch in the optic disc rim.
• The cup–disc ratio increases over time due to nerve fibre loss on the retinal surface, which come together to form the rim of the optic nerve head. As the rim thins, the cup size relative to the disc enlarges. This may happen asymmetrically between the two eyes.
• The cup–disc ratio change denotes anatomical or structural damage. This has functional effects that manifest as defects in the visual field, typically arcuate scotomas and nasal steps. The patient does not usually notice these defects which are picked up on automated visual field testing and analysis.

Treatment

• Aim to reduce the IOP; medically (topical drop treatment is most commonly used), with laser treatments or surgically. (See Chapter 41 for details.)
• Patients with established disease require lifelong follow-up.

Acute angle-closure glaucoma (AACG) (Figure 39.4)

This is an ophthalmic emergency. Patients with AACG can go blind if there is a delay in diagnosis and management. If it occurs in one eye, the fellow eye is also at risk.

Risk factors

• Age: AACG is more common in elderly patients, particularly those with significant increase in anteroposterior size of their lens as their cataract develops.
• Race: angle-closure glaucoma is the commonest glaucoma in Chinese.

• Hypermetropia (longsightedness).

Symptoms

• Sudden-onset headache with a painful red eye, nausea, vomiting, halos around lights and decreased vision.

Signs

• Reduced visual acuity.
• Mid-dilated fixed pupil on the affected side.
• Hazy view of the iris and pupil in the affected eye from a cloudy oedematous cornea.
• Red eye.
• Rapidly raised IOP over a few hours. The speed of IOP rise in AACG is important. In POAG there may be high but asymptomatic IOP because the IOP has risen gradually over a period of months.
• Closed angle on gonioscopy.

Treatment

• Urgent treatment to reduce the IOP and prevent recurrences.
• Medical treatment with intravenous acetazolamide, a powerful suppressor of aqueous production, then oral Diamox to maintain the effect.
• Topical aqueous suppressors (e.g. beta-blockers and alpha-agonists).
• Pilocarpine drops to constrict both pupils which alters the iris and ciliary body configuration and opens the drainage angles.
• Prevent further attacks with Yag laser peripheral iridotomy (PI) or surgical iridectomy.
• Treat the second eye prophylactically.
• If PIs are not sufficient, specialist management is required and may involve peripheral iris laser or surgical lens extraction.

Secondary glaucoma

• Many eye conditions can cause a secondary rise in IOP with optic nerve damage (e.g. trauma, inflammation, complicated cataract surgery and rubeosis).
• Treat the cause where possible (e.g. PRP for rubeosis or steroid drops for inflammation and reducing the IOP).

Chronic angle-closure glaucoma

Unlike AACG, the speed of IOP rise is slower in CACG. CACG occurs in small eyes where there is asymptomatic adhesion between the peripheral iris and the cornea progressively occluding the drainage angle. Initial treatment usually involves a laser PI.

Congenital glaucoma or infantile glaucoma

Uncommon, either unilateral or bilateral, primary or associated with ocular malformations or systemic syndromes (e.g. Sturge–Weber syndrome). It should be suspected in an infant or child with persistent watering photophobic eyes and in cases of clouding of the cornea.

Signs

• Large eye, or buphthalmos.
• Wider than average corneal diameters.
• Reduced vision.
• Clouding of the cornea.
• Linear tears in Descemet's membrane (known as Haabs' striae).
• Raised IOP.

Treatment

Congenital and juvenile glaucoma requires subspecialist management.

KEY POINTS

• Normal range of intraocular pressure is 10–21 mmHg.
• Primary open-angle glaucoma is the commonest form.
• Acute angle-closure glaucoma occurs in older persons and is usually painful.

Figure 40.1 Scanning laser ophthalmoscopy (SLO) picture to monitor disc changes: showing progressive disc cupping with a thinning neural rim, especially inferiorly

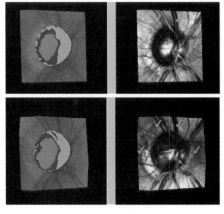

Figure 40.2 Goldmann tonometry. (a) At slit lamp, (b) the tonometer touches the anaesthezied cornea and (c) two half rings are seen and approximated to read pressure in millimetres of mercury (mmHg)

(a)

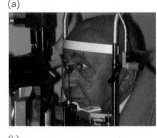

(b)

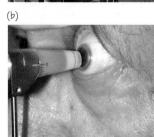

(c)

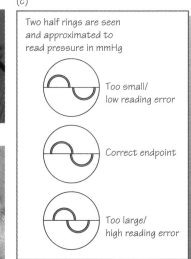

Two half rings are seen and approximated to read pressure in mmHg

Too small/ low reading error

Correct endpoint

Too large/ high reading error

Figure 40.3 (a) Automated visual field testing and (b) Humphrey analyser shows a progressing field defect in the superior arcuate

(a)

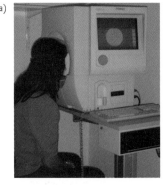

(b)

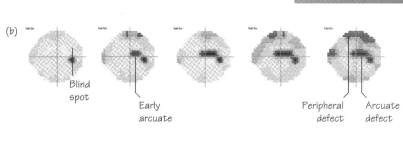

Blind spot

Early arcuate

Peripheral defect

Arcuate defect

Figure 40.4 (a) A four-mirror Zeiss goniolens, (b) a gonioscopic view of anterior chamber angle, (c) a gonio lens to allow view of drainage angle, (d) a Magna View lens and (e) structures seen in angle

(a)

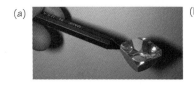

(b)

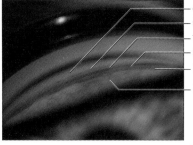

Cornea
Schwalbe's white line
Trabecular meshwork
Scleral spur
Iris root (ciliary body)
Iris

(c)

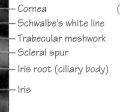

Observation

(d)

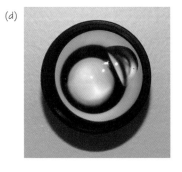

(e)

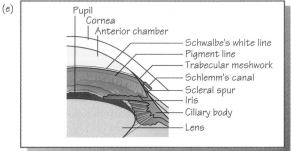

Pupil
Cornea
Anterior chamber
Schwalbe's white line
Pigment line
Trabecular meshwork
Schlemm's canal
Scleral spur
Iris
Ciliary body
Lens

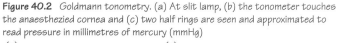

Ophthalmology at a Glance, Second Edition. Jane Olver, Lorraine Cassidy, Gurjeet Jutley, and Laura Crawley. © 2014 Jane Olver, Lorraine Cassidy, Gurjeet Jutley and Laura Crawley. Published 2014 by John Wiley & Sons, Ltd. Companion Website: www.ataglanceseries.com/ophthal

Aim

Understand how glaucoma is diagnosed.

History taking

Apart from acute angle-closure glaucoma, most forms of glaucoma are asymptomatic until very advanced optic nerve damage has occurred. A positive family history of glaucoma and myopia are important risk factors in the history.

Clinical examination

- **Visual acuity:** Reduced by advanced chronic glaucoma damage or acute angle-closure glaucoma.
- **Ocular examination:**
  - Slit lamp examination for anterior segment abnormalities associated with glaucoma.
  - Detailed assessment of optic disc. Ideally, the optic disc is photographed (conventional or with 3D scanning laser ophthalmoscope; Figure 40.1) to enable the detection of progression.
- **Intraocular (IOP) measurement:** Using a Goldmann applanation tonometer (Figure 40.2). Measures force needed to flatten a defined area of cornea. This force corresponds to IOP, measured in millimetres of mercury. Note: normal tension glaucoma has normal-range IOP.
- **Visual field testing:** Usually assessed with automated perimetry to allow efficient repeat testing to detect progression. Classic defect is arcuate scotoma (Figure 40.3).
- **Gonioscopy:** Used to assess the anterior chamber angle (Figure 40.4). This cannot be viewed directly, so a gonioprism lens is used—the optics of which allow visualization of the angle between the cornea and iris.

Glaucoma is diagnosed if a glaucomatous optic neuropathy (typical optic disc and field changes) is found to be present. Other parts of the examination help classify the glaucoma so that appropriate treatment can be given.

- **Pachymetry:** Used to measure the thickness of the cornea. Average corneal thickness is 540–560 μm. Thinner than average corneas in the presence of high IOP are a risk factor for glaucomatous damage.

> **TIP**
>
> - Do not rely on IOP measurement alone for the diagnosis and monitoring of glaucoma as the IOP may be in the normal range, yet disc and field changes may be present.

Monitoring

Once a patient has been diagnosed and started on treatment, the same techniques are used at regular intervals to assess for progression. Finding the correct treatment to prevent progression depends on these same examination techniques.

Screening

Most forms of glaucoma are asymptomatic until very advanced optic nerve damage has occurred. Treatment at this stage is often too late, so glaucoma patients may be actively sought out from the community (i.e. screened). This is usually done by opticians, who assess IOP, visual fields and optic disc appearance. Two main groups of people are screened:
- People with a family history of glaucoma, especially primary open-angle glaucoma.
- All people over 40 will have IOP measured at a sight test.

If an abnormality suggestive of glaucoma is detected in this screening process, the person is referred to the hospital ophthalmology department.

Problems of glaucoma screening

- People are missed if they do not attend opticians.
- False positives are common because the initial assessment of field and disc is difficult.

> **WARNING**
>
> ▶ Some patients have primary open angle glaucoma with normal IOP.

> **KEY POINTS**
>
> - Glaucoma screening by opticians helps detect primary open-angle glaucoma.
> - A family history of primary open-angle glaucoma is a risk factor for developing glaucoma.
> - Automated visual field analysis is used to monitor visual field progression.

Glaucoma surgery

Glaucoma or drainage surgery is indicated when there is progression of glaucoma not controlled by medication or laser. Laser iridotomy prevents acute angle-closure attacks

Note: See also Appendix 3: Pharmacological intraocular pressure (IOP) lowering agents – mechanism of action and side effects

Laser treatments

Figure 41.1 Peripheral iridotomy

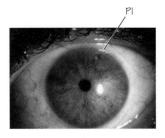

PI

Figure 41.2 Selective laser trabeculoplasty treatment

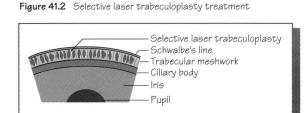

Selective laser trabeculoplasty
Schwalbe's line
Trabecular meshwork
Ciliary body
Iris
Pupil

Figure 41.3 Cyclodiode

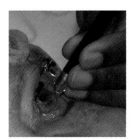

Surgical treatments

Figure 41.4 Trabeculectomy. (a) Diffuse bleb and (b) thin-walled bleb. These are at risk of infection and usually require revision surgery. (c) Schematic diagrams showing the bleb in relation to eye anatomy

(a) Diffuse bleb

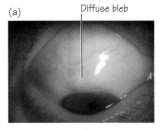

(b)

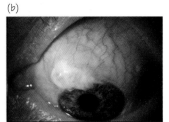

(c)

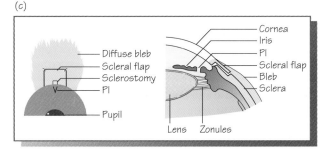

Diffuse bleb
Scleral flap
Sclerostomy
PI
Pupil

Cornea
Iris
PI
Scleral flap
Bleb
Sclera
Lens Zonules

Figure 41.5 Leaking wound–a positive Siedel test (trabeculectomy bleb leak)

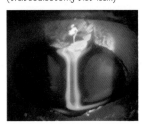

Figure 41.6 Drainage devices and tubes

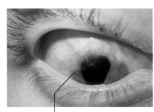

Tube in anterior chamber

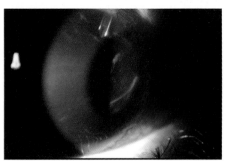

Ophthalmology at a Glance, Second Edition. Jane Olver, Lorraine Cassidy, Gurjeet Jutley, and Laura Crawley. © 2014 Jane Olver, Lorraine Cassidy, Gurjeet Jutley and Laura Crawley. Published 2014 by John Wiley & Sons, Ltd. Companion Website: www.ataglanceseries.com/ophthal

Aims

- Understand the aims of medical, laser and surgical treatment.
- Be familiar with different classes of drugs used to treat primary open-angle glaucoma.
- Manage a case of acute angle-closure glaucoma.

Treatment goal: To preserve the patient's sight throughout his or her lifetime with minimum side effects

- Treat to lower intraocular pressure (IOP). This is currently the only modifiable risk factor and is the main aim of glaucoma therapy. Lowering IOP can be achieved by reducing aqueous production (inflow) or enhancing aqueous drainage (outflow.) There is no single target IOP that will be appropriate for all patients. Treatment and target IOP are tailored to each patient's findings—the patient's presenting IOP, visual field, optic disc appearance and type of glaucoma.
- Ensure good ocular perfusion. Prevent arteriosclerosis, treat vasospasm and minimize low blood pressure (nocturnal dips).

Medical therapy

Most patients with primary open-angle glaucoma (POAG) can be managed with topical drop treatment. The aim of medical treatment is to prevent the progression of disc cupping or visual field defect. Pharmacological modulation of carbonic anhydrase, adenosine triphosphatases and adrenoreceptors located in the nonpigmented ciliary epithelium can reduce aqueous production and thus lower IOP. Similarly, pharmacological modulation of adrenoreceptors and prostanoid receptors located in the trabecular meshwork or ciliary body can increase aqueous outflow through both pathways and lower IOP. Pharmacological treatments to lower IOP have improved dramatically. The improved efficacy and tolerability of these drugs are in part responsible for the reduction in the number of glaucoma operations carried out since the 1990s. The primary treatment agents for this condition are summarized in Appendix 3, 'Pharmacological IOP-lowering agents', which can be found at the back of the book for easy reference.

Laser treatment

- **Bypass pupil block—peripheral iridectomy (Figure 41.1)**: this is the treatment of choice to prevent angle-closure glaucoma or after an acute attack has been broken with medical treatment. A YAG (yttrium–aluminium–garnet) laser hole in the peripheral iris allows aqueous flow from the posterior to anterior chamber.
- **Enhance aqueous outflow—trabeculoplasty (Figure 41.2)**: laser to the trabecular meshwork enhances aqueous outflow. Several different lasers can be used to apply this treatment, including argon laser trabeculoplasty (ALT), selective laser trabeculoplasty (SLT) and micropulse diode laser trabeculoplasty (MDLT).
- **Decrease aqueous production—cyclodestruction**: laser to the ciliary body reduces aqueous production. This can be done through the sclera (trans-scleral cyclodiode; Figure 41.3) or endoscopically (endocyclophotocoagulation).

Surgical treatment

- Peripheral iridectomy. Used in acute angle-closure glaucoma (AACG) when laser is not possible.
- Trabeculectomy (Figure 41.4). A trabeculectomy creates a fistula between the anterior chamber of the eye and the subconjunctival space to allow controlled release of aqueous. It is still the most commonly performed surgery for POAG worldwide. A small full-thickness scleral hole is covered by a half-thickness scleral flap. Fluid flows from the anterior chamber, passes under the flap and drains under the conjunctiva. The scleral flap and conjunctiva can scar, thus reducing the flow and limiting the effectiveness of the operation. Antimetabolites such as mitomycin C and 5-fluorouracil are used to modulate the healing response and improve success rates. Risks include cataract, hypotony, infection and bleb leakage (Figure 41.5).
- Drainage devices or tubes (Figure 41.6). Silicone tube inserted into the anterior chamber and connected to a scleral sutured plate to drain aqueous.
- Deep sclerectomy. A section of the sclera and the roof of Schlemm's canal are excised. No penetration into the anterior chamber is required.
- Viscocanalostomy and canaloplasty. This is a deep sclerectomy with additional mechanical opening or stretching of Schlemm's canal.
- Drainage angle implants. Small, snorkel-like tube implants placed directly into the drainage angle of the eye (iStent®). This is usually combined with cataract surgery.

Treatment of AACG

AACG requires medical, laser and surgical treatment. Immediate treatment is medical to reduce the IOP and to break the attack of angle closure.

- Intravenous carbonic anhydrase inhibitor (acetazolamide, 500 mg) is used to reduce the production of aqueous fluid.
- Oral acetazolamide is often required for ongoing aqueous suppression for 1–2 days.
- Pilocarpine is usually instilled in both eyes. This helps to break the acute attack and reduce the risk of further attacks, particularly in the fellow eye.
- Topical agents help reduce IOP (e.g. timolol and iopidine).
- Perform bilateral peripheral iridotomies as soon as possible.
- Rarely, lens extraction or trabeculectomy is required.

KEY POINTS

- Most POAG patients are treated medically, typically with once-daily prostaglandin analogues or once-daily combination drops of prostaglandin analogues and beta-blockers.
- Trabeculectomy lowers the IOP by draining the aqueous into a small subconjunctival bleb from where the fluid is reabsorbed.
- Surgery is indicated for disease progression in POAG.

Figure 42.1 Anatomy of a retina. (a) Cross-sectional anatomy and (b) when viewed with an ophthalmoscope

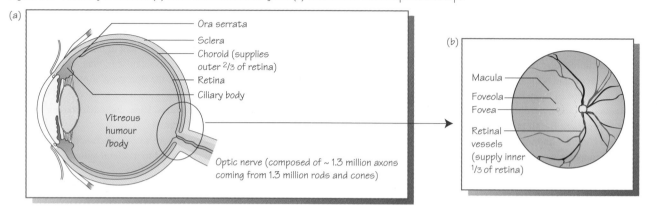

(a)

Ora serrata

Sclera

Choroid (supplies outer 2/3 of retina)

Retina

Ciliary body

Vitreous humour /body

Optic nerve (composed of ~ 1.3 million axons coming from 1.3 million rods and cones)

(b)

Macula

Foveola

Fovea

Retinal vessels (supply inner 1/3 of retina)

Figure 42.2 Posterior vitreous detachment (PVD). (a) Cross-sectional appearance and (b) when viewed with an ophthalmoscope

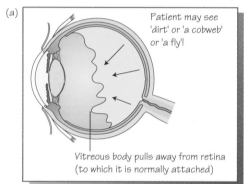

(a)

Patient may see 'dirt' or 'a cobweb' or 'a fly'!

Vitreous body pulls away from retina (to which it is normally attached)

(b)

On ophthalmoscopy:

May see Weiss' ring floating in front of disc

Posterior vitreous detachment (PVD)
The vitreous gel 'jelly' separates from the posterior retina. This also causes 'floaters' such as a Weiss ring and is more common in older patients and myopics

Floaters
More noticeable on a sunny clear day against a blue sky, or white snow, or a white wall/ceiling. They can be particularly annoying when patients find that they get in the way of reading. They are common at any age.
NB many people have floaters

WARNING
Patients with PVD should be warned of the risk of retinal tear and detachment – should they notice a sudden shower of floaters or new flashing lights or a shadow at the edge of their vision, they should seek an urgent ophthalmological opinion

Figure 42.3 Rhegmatogenous retinal detachment

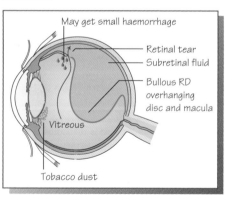

May get small haemorrhage

Retinal tear

Subretinal fluid

Bullous RD overhanging disc and macula

Vitreous

Tobacco dust

WARNING
If the macula is detached there is a risk of permanent visual impairment

Figure 42.4 Tractional retinal detachment

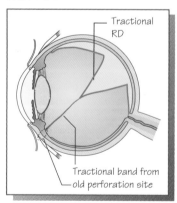

Tractional RD

Tractional band from old perforation site

Figure 42.5 Appearance of a retinal detachment. (a) Macula on retinal detachment and (b) large retinal tear and detachment

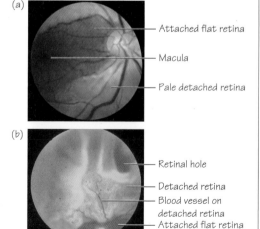

(a)

Attached flat retina

Macula

Pale detached retina

(b)

Retinal hole

Detached retina

Blood vessel on detached retina

Attached flat retina

Optic disc

Ophthalmology at a Glance, Second Edition. Jane Olver, Lorraine Cassidy, Gurjeet Jutley, and Laura Crawley. © 2014 Jane Olver, Lorraine Cassidy, Gurjeet Jutley and Laura Crawley. Published 2014 by John Wiley & Sons, Ltd. Companion Website: www.ataglanceseries.com/ophthal

Aims

- Understand the significance of eye floaters.
- Describe the types of retinal detachment.

The retina detaches if it has a hole or tear from high myopia, an inherent retinal weakness, or trauma. If part of the peripheral retina is detached, this is perceived as a peripheral vision shadow. If the macula is detached, central vision is very blurred (Figure 42.1).

Floaters and photopsia (flashing lights)

Floaters and flashes are common and alarming. The underlying cause ranges from the trivial to sight threatening.

Refer to an ophthalmologist if: new flurry of floaters (above and beyond the background basal level) or new flashing lights.

Floaters are caused by:

- Cells: in anterior, intermediate or posterior uveitis
- Blood: in vitreous haemorrhage
- Collapsed vitreous: common with age or axial myopia.

Photopsia are caused by stimulation of retinal photoreceptors by mechanical forces, simulating light activation:

- Retinal tears or detachments
- Detached vitreous gel tugging on the retina when abnormal adhesions are present.

Posterior vitreous detachment (PVD)

(Figure 42.2)

The vitreous gel pulls away or separates from the retina and collapses. A PVD is perceived as a floating cobweb, ring or tadpole, which moves with eye movement, worse against a white or clear background.

Aetiology

- Eye or head trauma or spontaneously with age or myopia greater than −6D.

Symptoms

- Photopsia; more noticeable in dim light.
- Floaters:
  - from a small amount of haemorrhage (which may occur with the PVD)
  - collapsed vitreous casts a shadow on the retina.

Natural history of floaters

The majority of floaters are self-limiting becoming less noticeable with time. Only a small proportion develop a retinal tear. In up to 15% of patients who present with an acute symptomatic PVD, the detaching vitreous pulls a hole in the retina, which can lead to a rhegmatogenous retinal detachment.

Management

- Indirect ophthalmoscopy with scleral indentation is used for mapping the retinal detachment.
- Laser treatment to seal a simple retinal tear with minimum or no sub-retinal fluid (SRF) and prevent retinal detachment (laser retinopexy).
- Reassure if no tear is found.

Retinal detachment (RD)

- An RD occurs when the retina is separated from the retinal pigment epithelium (RPE) by SRF.
- Once the retina has been separated from its blood supply, the photoreceptors slowly degenerate, becoming permanently non-functional.
- A RD is surgically reattached to regain vision.
- If the RD does not involve the macula (macula 'on' RD) and the vision is still good, surgery is urgent within 24 h particularly in superior detachments as gravity encourages it to track down toward the macula and threaten vision.

Aetiology

There are three types of RD, and each has a different aetiology:

- Rhegmatogenous RD (Figure 42.3): a full-thickness tear in the retina allows liquid vitreous into the space between the retina and the RPE. High myopia increases the risk.
- Exudative RD: some inflammatory or neoplastic conditions lead to serous exudation from leaky blood vessels beneath the retina (in the absence of a retinal break or hole).
- Tractional RD (Figure 42.4): fibrous or vascular membranes growing abnormally in the vitreous (e.g. in patients with fibrosis following proliferative diabetic retinopathy) contract and pull the retina away from the RPE.
- Solid RD: rarely, a tumour such as a malignant melanoma originating in the choroid under the retina can elevate the retina. This can metastasize and needs urgent referral to a specialist ophthalmic oncologist in a specialist centre for management.

Symptoms

Rhegmatogenous RD presents with:

- Photopsia ± floaters.
- This is followed by a gradual blurring or loss of vision, which may start off as a shadow in the peripheral visual field.
- SRF under the macula, (macula 'off' RD), causes blurred vision.
- Other types of RD present with reduced vision.

Signs (Figure 42.5)

- Visual acuity (VA) normal when the macula is on.
- Reduced VA be due to macular SRF or from a bullous RD in front of the macula.
- 'Tobacco dust' visible in the anterior vitreous represent red blood cells and/or RPE cells that have migrated into the vitreous through the tear. Tobacco dust indicates a retinal tear and the need for referral to a retinal surgery ophthalmologist for further evaluation.
- Intraocular pressure may be reduced.

Examination

Slit lamp examination for tobacco dust and with a three-mirror contact lens to detect the retinal tear and determine whether laser or surgery required.

Indirect ophthalmoscopy with scleral indentation assists viewing the RD.

Complications

- If the RD involves the macular area, recovery of vision is poor.
- Recurrent RD carries the risk of subretinal membrane and secondary tractional detachment.

Surgical management

- Rhegmatogenous RD: reattachment: laser, cryotherapy plus explant or internal surgery with vitrectomy.
- Exudative and solid RD: establish and treat the cause.
- Tractional RD: relieve traction.

In all types of vitreo-retinal surgery, an oil or gas may be used and patient posturing required post-operative.

> ### KEY POINTS
>
> - PVD results in floaters: look for a retinal tear.
> - Sub-retinal fluid gets under the retina through a tear and lifts the sensory retina off the retinal pigment epithelium, causing a detachment.
> - Some RDs do not have tears but are exudative, tractional or solid.

Figure 43.1 Chorio-retinal anatomy

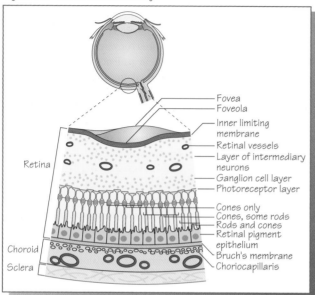

Fovea
Foveola
Inner limiting membrane
Retinal vessels
Layer of intermediary neurons
Ganglion cell layer
Photoreceptor layer
Cones only
Cones, some rods
Rods and cones
Retinal pigment epithelium
Bruch's membrane
Choriocapillaris

Retina
Choroid
Sclera

Figure 43.2 Posterior pole and retina. (a) Normal posterior pole and (b) topography

(a)

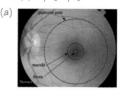

- Posterior pole area centralis (5–6 mm)
- Macula fovea (1.5 mm)
- Fovea foveola (350 μm)

(b)

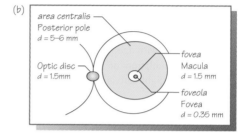

area centralis
Posterior pole
d = 5–6 mm
Optic disc
d = 1.5mm
fovea
Macula
d = 1.5 mm
foveola
Fovea
d = 0.35 mm

Note: See also Appendix 2: The layers of the retina

Figure 43.3 Ocular coherence tomography. (a) Optic nerve and (b) macula

(a) (b)

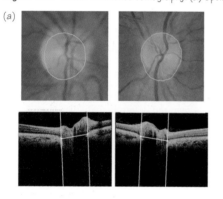

Figure 43.5 Fluorescein angiography – normal macula

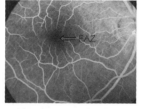

i) Retinal vessels imaged with fluorescein angiogram showing loss of capillary network at foveal avascular zone (FAZ)

KEY POINTS

- Fluorescein angiography provides fine detail of the retinal structures and vessels
- Indocyanine green provides information about the choroidal vessels

Figure 43.6 Indocyanine green angiography – the same normal macula as Figure 43.5

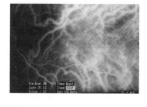

ii) Choroidal vessels imaged. Indocyanine green angiogram (ICGA) showing rich choroidal blood supply at macula

Figure 43.4 Dye physics. (a) Disc report and (b) macula report

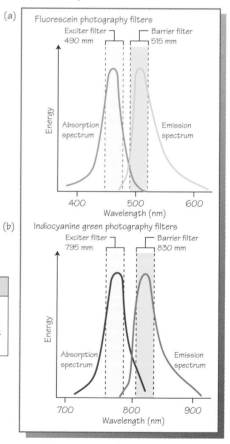

(a) Fluorescein photography filters

Exciter filter 490 mm
Barrier filter 515 mm
Absorption spectrum
Emission spectrum
Energy
400 500 600
Wavelength (nm)

(b) Indiocyanine green photography filters

Exciter filter 795 mm
Barrier filter 830 mm
Absorption spectrum
Emission spectrum
Energy
700 800 900
Wavelength (nm)

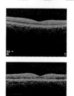

Ophthalmology at a Glance, Second Edition. Jane Olver, Lorraine Cassidy, Gurjeet Jutley, and Laura Crawley. © 2014 Jane Olver, Lorraine Cassidy,
104 Gurjeet Jutley and Laura Crawley. Published 2014 by John Wiley & Sons, Ltd. Companion Website: www.ataglanceseries.com/ophthal

The ability to image the microstructure of the retina and choroid has significantly altered the way we appreciate and treat retinal disease.

Aims
• Know the anatomy of the choroid and retina.
• Identify the main priorities of medical retinal disease.
• Know the methods of retinal imaging and the appropriate use of a particular imaging system.
• Understand the need for more than one modality of imaging.

Retinal and choroidal anatomy
(Figure 43.1)
Knowledge of retinal anatomy and physiology is vital to accurately interpret retinal images.
• **Choroid**: a fenestrated capillary-rich layer which supplies oxygen and micronutrients to the retinal pigment epithelium and the outer one-third of the neurosensory retina. The capillary layer is the choriocapillaris.
• **Retinal pigment epithelium (RPE)**: a monolayer of pigmented cells between the neurosensory retina and Bruch's membrane. Tight junctions exclude large molecules and form the outer part of the blood retinal barrier.
• **Bruch's membrane**: an acellular layer between the choroid and RPE, which does not form a significant part of the blood–retinal barrier.
• **Neurosensory retina**: includes photoreceptors, ganglion cells and their axons (nerve fibre layer), other neurons (e.g. bipolar cells) and glial cells (e.g. Müller cells).
• **Retinal arteries, capillaries and veins**: non-fenestrated vessels forming the inner blood–retinal barrier.
• **Foveal avascular zone**: an approximately 0.045 mm zone in which retinal capillaries are absent.

Medical retinal disease priorities
The management of medical retinal disease has been revolutionized as a result of developments in retinal imaging, the advent of molecular genetics and new treatment modalities.

Retinal imaging modalities, together with psychophysical and electrophysiological evaluation, are very valuable in diagnosing disorders of the retina, RPE and choroid.

Imaging
Fundus camera (Figure 43.2)
• A high-resolution digital fundus camera can be used to document baseline retinal findings and track disease progression, and for screening (e.g. for diabetic retinopathy) and clinical studies. Colour fundus photography and fluorescein and indocyanine green angiography are used to image the retina and surrounding structures. Digital images allow rapid diagnosis and review, and are electronically transferred; they are useful for telemedicine.
Optical coherence tomography (OCT) (Figure 43.3)
This is non-invasive diagnostic imaging analogous to an ultrasound B scan except that light and not sound is used; a higher resolution is therefore obtainable. A highly coherent light source is used to scan the retina and produces high-resolution, cross-sectional, three-dimensional (3D) images. Used for assessing retinal thickness, retinal oedema and optic nerve head imaging in glaucoma, and for assessing macula pathology. OCT is becoming the most commonly performed retinal imaging. Fluorescein angiography can be done using an OCT machine. Also see Appendix 4 for full OCT reports.
Dyes used in imaging (Figure 43.4)
• **Fluorescein**: sodium fluorescein is an orange dye excited by a blue light to emit a yellow-green light. It is a small molecule, only 80% bound to blood proteins, which diffuses freely through the choriocapillaris, Bruch's membrane, optic nerve and sclera.
• **Indocyanine green (ICG)**: this is a green dye, which when excited by a near-infrared light emits a near-infrared light. It is almost 100% protein bound, so it only leaks slowly through the fenestrated capillaries of the choriocapillaris.

Fundus fluorescein angiogram (FFA) (Figure 43.5)
This is a sequence of fundus images taken immediately after sodium fluorescein dye is injected into a peripheral vein. The fundus is illuminated by a blue light, causing the fluorescein molecules to fluoresce in the yellow-green spectrum. Barrier filters block reflected blue light so that only yellow-green (i.e. fluorescent) light is transmitted to the film or digital camera. A detailed 3D view of the retina and of the level of fluorescence can be achieved by using a stereoscopic viewing device or computer software. FFA is good for viewing retinal detail.

Indocyanine green angiography (ICGA) (Figure 43.6)
Near-infrared fluorescence is recorded with infrared film or, more commonly, with a digital camera, after the injection of ICG into a peripheral vein. Light of this wavelength has better penetration of red or brown pigments (e.g. melanin in RPE cells or sub-retinal blood). ICGA is useful in investigating choroidal disease (e.g. choroidal neo-vascularization and choroidal tumours).

Confocal scanning laser ophthalmoscope (SLO)
This is a fundus camera using a low-power scanning laser for illumination at different focal planes in the retina to produce tomographic images.

Terms used when describing fluorescein angiograms
• **Hyperfluorescence**: increased fluorescence relative to other structures; seen as black on white if negative film is used and white on black with digital photography
• **Hypofluorescence**: reduced fluorescence relative to other structures (e.g. due to blocked fluorescence or decreased vascular perfusion)
• **Window defect**: increased choroidal fluorescence seen through a window of attenuated RPE (e.g. geographic atrophy or laser scars)
• **Blocked fluorescence**: masking of fluorescence by opacity anterior to it (e.g. sub-retinal haemorrhage)
• **Fluorescein leakage**: characteristic of conditions in which the outer (RPE) or inner (retinal vasculature) blood–retinal barrier is disrupted
• **Autofluorescence**: fluorescence occurring without the injection of fluorescein dye.

Side effects of fluorescein and indocyanine green		
	Fluorescein	Indocyanine green (ICG)
Contraindications		
Absolute	Fluorescein allergy	ICG, iodine or shellfish allergy
	History of severe allergies	History of severe allergies
Relative	Asthma	Asthma
	Ischaemic heart disease	Ischaemic heart disease
	Previous allergic reaction	Previous allergic reaction
	Renal failure (use lower dose)	Liver failure
Adverse effects	Skin discolouration	Mild to moderate 0.35% (e.g. hypotension)
	Nausea 3–5%	Severe 0.05% (e.g. anaphylaxis)
	Allergy 0.5–1%	

Microanatomy

Photoreceptors: Rods: for vision in dim light (shades of black and white) and motion vision. Cones: for vision in bright light (high resolution and colour). Rods predominate outside the fovea, cones are most dense at the fovea. **Retinal Pigment Epithelium (RPE):** Single layer of cells with an important role in the turnover and support of photoreceptor outer-segments and formation of photosensitive pigments. Forms the *blood-retinal barrier*. **Bruch's Membrane:** Separates the RPE from choriocapillaris. See Chapter 40

Definitions

Dystrophy: Inherited disorder
Photophobia: Painful sensation in bright light
Nyctalopia: Poor or lack of vision in the dark
Phenotype: Clinical characterization including symptoms (e.g. photophobia, nyctalopia), fundus appearance and functional assessment

Inherited retinal dystrophies

Classification of age related macular degeneration (AMD)

Dry AMD

Figure 44.4 Age-related maculopathy. (a) Histopathology and (b) colour fundus picture of soft confluent Drusen at macula
Figure 44.4a courtesy of Victor Chong

(a)

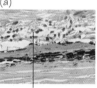

Soft Drusen

(b)

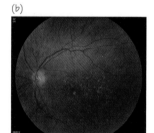

Figure 44.6 Colour fundus photograph of right eye showing a large area of geographical atrophy at the macula

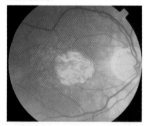

Figure 44.7 Widespread drusen and neovascular membrane

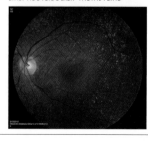

Table 44.1 Risk factors for age-related macular degeneration

- Age
- Female sex
- Smoking
- Light iris colour
- Pseudophakia
- Hypermetropia
- Hypertension, and cardiovascular and cerebrovascular disease
- Family history: polymorphism in the gene coding complement factor H

Figure 44.1 Central dystrophy: best dystrophy

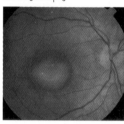

Figure 44.2 Mixed dystrophy: cone rod

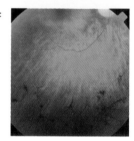

Figure 44.3 Peripheral dystrophy: retinitis pigmentosa with intraretinal mid-peripheral bone spicule pigmentation

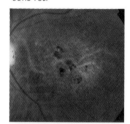

See also Appendix 5: Important clinical trials in AMD

Wet AMD

Figure 44.5 Choroidal neovascularization (CNV)

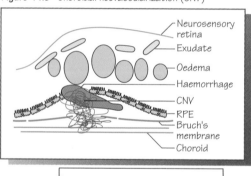

- Neurosensory retina
- Exudate
- Oedema
- Haemorrhage
- CNV
- RPE
- Bruch's membrane
- Choroid

Figure 44.8 Classic CNV

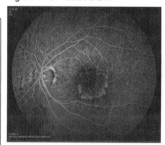

Figure 44.9 Occult CNV

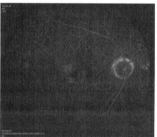

KEY POINTS

- Inherited retinal disorders are common, accurate early diagnosis is important for prognosis and genetic counselling. No cures are available but clinical trials of novel therapies are being conductd
- AMD is the leading cause of blindness in industrialized countries
- Sudden-onset central distortion and blurring may be treatable CNV

Improved imaging techniques including high-resolution optical coherence tomography (OCT) and the availability of multiple intravitreal treatments (see Appendix 4) and novel interventions such as gene and stem cell therapies has revolutionized the management of inherited retinal disorders and age-related macular degeneration (AMD). Inherited retinal disorders most commonly present in childhood or early adulthood whereas AMD is most common in older adults. AMD is the most common cause of visual loss in the western world. In the UK, inherited retinal disease is the second commonest cause of visual loss in childhood and the commonest cause in the working-age population.

Aims
- Appreciate the types of inherited retinal degeneration.
- Know the significance of early central visual symptoms of neovascular age-related macular degeneration (nAMD) and refer promptly for early treatment.
- Be aware of the range of treatment options and increasing clinical trials for patients with inherited retinal degeneration and AMD.

Children and young adults
Inherited retinal disorders
- Divided into predominantly stationary conditions (cone or rod dysfunction syndromes e.g. achromatopsia and congenital stationary night blindness, respectively)—or progressive disorders (retinal dystrophies—rod-cone dystrophies, cone-rod dystrophies, and chorioretinal dystrophies).
- Stationary disorders tend to present at birth or early infancy whereas Progressive disorders often present in the first or second decades.
- Clinical and genetic variability in inherited retinal disease within and between families severity, age of onset, and rate of progression.
- Retinal dystrophies Stargardt disease, Best's disease (Figure 44.1), North Carolina macular dystrophy cone–rod dystrophy (Figure 44.2).
- Retinitis pigmentosa (RP) (Figure 44.3) is a rod-cone dystrophy incidence of approximately 1 in 3000. Early features due to loss of rod function are night blindness and progressive peripheral visual field loss, with later loss of cone function resulting in central visual loss. Full-field electroretinograms in the early stages show a greater reduction in the responses of the rod system than the cone system, with often unrecordable ERGs at later stages. Characteristic retinal findings: optic disc pallor, retinal vessel attenuation and widespread bone-spicule retinal pigmentation. RP is most commonly isolated (non-syndromic) but can be associated with systemic disease (syndromic RP), including Usher syndrome (RP with deafness) and Kearns–Sayre syndrome (RP with ophthalmoplegia, ataxia and cardiac conduction defects).
- Genetic counselling, advice on prognosis and increasingly molecular genetic testing are important in the management of these disorders.
- There are no proven cures for inherited retinal disorders—we are in an era of increasing clinical trials of gene therapy, stem cell therapy, artificial vision, and neuroprotective and pharmacological approaches. Further information from www.clinicaltrials.gov and the research section on the website of Retinitis Pigmentosa Fighting Blindness.
- Management: ensuring appropriate spectacle correction, low visual aids, providing educational and social support, and visual impairment certification. The use of vitamin A in RP is controversial with most authorities no longer recommending its use. Patients with Stargardt disease should not take Vitamin A as it is likely to be harmful. Patients are advised to not smoke, have a healthy balanced diet rich in green vegetables (lutein containing), and to avoid excessive exposure to bright sunlight including wearing sunglasses with good ultra-violet light blocking properties.

Older adults
Age-related macular degeneration
AMD is the commonest cause of blindness in the Western world. See Table 44.1 for the associated risk factors; two main forms of AMD occur: dry and wet; tobacco smoking is the main modifiable risk factor; genetic risk factors—consistent with an inflammatory basis to AMD, with complement factor H (*CFH*) and *C3* genes implicated in the pathogenesis of AMD. Non-complement factor associated genes include *ARMS2/HTRA1*; other significant risk factors: family history of AMD (OR = 3.95: CI 1.35–11.54), race. AMD is more common in whites.

Pathology
- Dry AMD accounts for 90% of cases. Oxidative stress and inflammation play an important role in pathogenesis. Retinal waste products including lipofuscin and A2-E accumulate in the RPE, impairing its function and resulting in photoreceptor and choriocapillaris damage. A2-E activates the complement system leading to localized chronic inflammation and further impairment of RPE function. Specific retinal changes include: localized collection of extracellular material (drusen) at Bruch's membrane (Figure 44.4), loss of RPE/photoreceptors, thickening of Bruch's membrane and choriocapillary atrophy.
- In 10% of patients, under the control of vascular endothelial growth factor (VEGF), blood vessels grow from the choroid, through Bruch's membrane and into the retina: wet AMD. These choroidal neovascular membranes (CNVMs; Figure 44.5) leak and cause scarring in the macula, hence causing irreversible loss of central vision.

Investigations
- Dry AMD—OCT and fundus autofluorescence imaging (FAF) can help document baseline disease severity and monitor progression.
- Wet AMD—Fundus fluorescein angiogram (FFA): important for diagnosis and assessment for treatment, identifying type of CNVM, and monitoring progress. OCT: detects macular oedema, subretinal fluid, pigment epithelial detachment (Figure 44.6 and 44.7). OCT measures disease progression and guide treatment. ICG: primarily used in diagnosis of idiopathic polypoidal choroidal vasculopathy with a role in diagnosis of retinal angiomatous proliferation.
- The two main types of wet AMD can be clearly diagnosed using FFA: early leakage of dye (classic neovascular membranes, Figure 44.8) and slower later leakage (occult CNVM; Figure 44.9).

Managing AMD
- Dry AMD: Lifestyle changes; cessation of smoking, protect eyes from excessive bright sunlight, healthy life style with weight reduction, well balanced diet high in natural antioxidants, green-leafy vegetables. Nutritional supplementation based upon AREDS / AREDS2 such as Ocuvite Lutein. Low visual assessment and aids. Amsler grid to monitor any new distortion (suggestive of conversion to the wet form of the disease). Future therapies include Complement system inhibitors: phase 2 trials underway.
- Wet AMD: The mainstay is intravitreal anti-VEGF which stop the stimulus for blood vessel growth and leakiness by injecting regular anti-VEGF drugs directly into the vitreous (through the pars plana and not damaging the neurosensory retina).
- We are guided for further repeat injections by serial assessments of visual function, retinal examination and OCT.
- Two principal NICE approved agents which are administered at differing intervals following the loading phase, ranibizumab and aflibercept. This provides disease stability is achieved in approximately 90% of patients, 3 line improvement in 30–40%.

Rehabilitation
Consider patients with wet or dry AMD for a Certificate of Visual Impairment.
- Entitlements: financial allowance, disabled person's parking badge, talking books and clocks etc; a home visit by a low-vision therapist to assess disability; initiate community care, social and/or voluntary services and contact with self-help groups.

Low-vision aids
- optical aids: magnifiers and telescopes
- non-optical aids: lighting, large-print books and bank statements.

Important trials (evidence-based medicine)
(See Appendix 5).

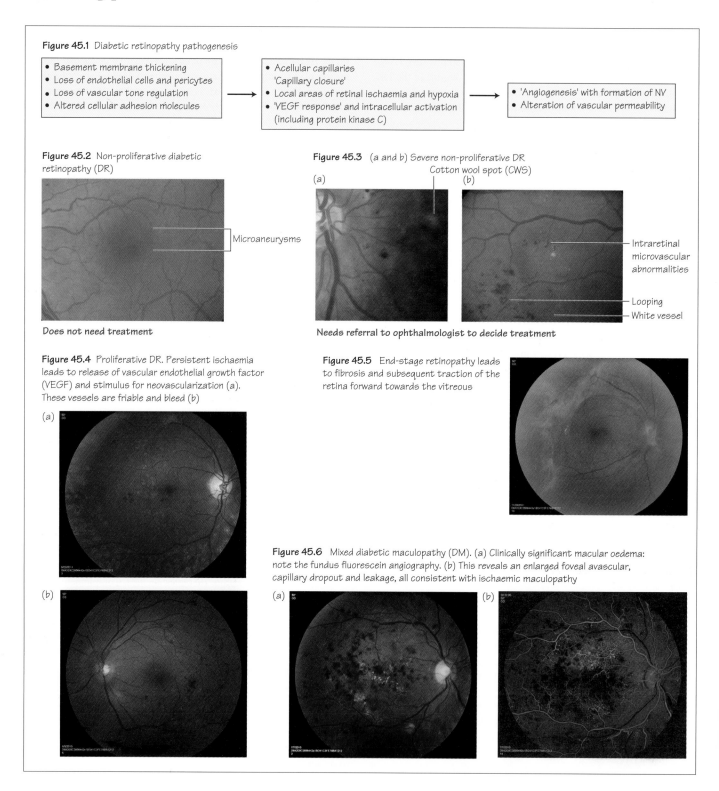

Figure 45.1 Diabetic retinopathy pathogenesis

- Basement membrane thickening
- Loss of endothelial cells and pericytes
- Loss of vascular tone regulation
- Altered cellular adhesion molecules

- Acellular capillaries 'Capillary closure'
- Local areas of retinal ischaemia and hypoxia
- 'VEGF response' and intracellular activation (including protein kinase C)

- 'Angiogenesis' with formation of NV
- Alteration of vascular permeability

Figure 45.2 Non-proliferative diabetic retinopathy (DR)

Microaneurysms

Does not need treatment

Figure 45.3 (a and b) Severe non-proliferative DR

Cotton wool spot (CWS)

(a)   (b)

Intraretinal microvascular abnormalities

Looping

White vessel

Needs referral to ophthalmologist to decide treatment

Figure 45.4 Proliferative DR. Persistent ischaemia leads to release of vascular endothelial growth factor (VEGF) and stimulus for neovascularization (a). These vessels are friable and bleed (b)

(a)

(b)

Figure 45.5 End-stage retinopathy leads to fibrosis and subsequent traction of the retina forward towards the vitreous

Figure 45.6 Mixed diabetic maculopathy (DM). (a) Clinically significant macular oedema: note the fundus fluorescein angiography. (b) This reveals an enlarged foveal avascular, capillary dropout and leakage, all consistent with ischaemic maculopathy

(a)   (b)

108 *Ophthalmology at a Glance*, Second Edition. Jane Olver, Lorraine Cassidy, Gurjeet Jutley, and Laura Crawley. © 2014 Jane Olver, Lorraine Cassidy, Gurjeet Jutley and Laura Crawley. Published 2014 by John Wiley & Sons, Ltd. Companion Website: www.ataglanceseries.com/ophthal

Aims
• Understand the pathogenesis and classification of diabetic retinopathy (DR) with relevance to visual loss.
• Understand the role of DR screening and the two-way communication between the community and the hospital.

Introduction
• DR is an important microvascular complication of diabetes mellitus.
• It is the leading cause of blindness in the working population in the developed world.
• The annual incidence of blindness from DR varies between 0.02% and 1%.
• An international standard classification of DR is essential for guidelines in screening, treatment protocols and research.

Pathology
One must think of DR as a continuum of disease, with a stepwise progression that leads to the various clinical manifestations (Figure 45.1). At the epicentre of this universe is ischaemia:
• Thickening of basement membranes, damage to and proliferation of endothelial cells, and increased platelet aggregation all lead to narrowed vessels.
• This causes ischaemia and leads to weakening of capillary walls, resulting in out-pouching of vessels.
• Further phosphorylation, glycosylation and disorganization of tight junctions, with a loss of pericytes, leads to breakdown of the inner blood–retinal barrier. Once enough damage to the vessel walls occur, they become leaky (large enough for extravasation of protein, lipids, red blood cells and fluid).
• Continual ischaemia leads to cotton wool spots and intra-retinal microvascular abnormalities (IRMAs).
• The retinal response to ischaemia is the release of vasogenic agents, including vascular endothelial growth factor (VEGF), which ultimately lead to neovascularization. Unfortunately, these new vessels are weak, friable and prone to haemorrhage. The endpoint is blindness from tractional retinal detachment or rubeotic glaucoma.

National screening committee classification of DR
• **R0** = no DR
• **R1 = mild non-proliferative or pre-proliferative DR disease (Figure 45.2)**
  ○ **Microaneurysms (MAs)**: out-pouching of retinal capillaries; may bleed, leak or become occluded.
  ○ **Haemorrhages**: bleeding from these leaky vessels, at various layers of the retina.
• **R2 = moderate and severe non-proliferative or pre-proliferative DR disease (Figure 45.3)**
  ○ **Hard exudates**: lipid components that are not easily removed by macrophages accumulate, often at the edge of the oedema, as characteristic yellowish lesions.

  ○ All of the following are indicative of established retinal ischaemia:
    ▪ **cotton wool spots (CWSs)**: micro-infarct of the retinal nerve fibre layer (NFL) causing a localized swelling of the NFL axon
    ▪ **venous beading**: venous irregularities, 'sausaging' and engorgement
    ▪ **IRMAs**: new vessels growing from the venous side of the bed of vessels, to compensate for an area of arterial non-perfusion.
• **R3 = proliferative retinopathy, pre-retinal fibrosis and tractional retinal detachment (Figures 45.4)**
  ○ **Retinal neovascularization and new vessels**: fragile new vessels grow outside the retina along the posterior surface of the vitreous. Changes in blood flow or traction on the new vessels, including posterior vitreous detachment, may cause them to haemorrhage into the vitreous cavity (vitreous haemorrhage; Figure 45.5). These vessels can grow as neovascularization of the optic disc (NVD) or as neovascularization elsewhere (NVE).
• **M0 = no maculopathy**
• **M1 = diabetic maculopathy (Figure 45.6)**
  ○ The macula is a circle centred around the fovea. The radius of the circle is the fovea to the disc margin. Clinically significant macular oedema (CSMO) involves or is near the fovea, and this is defined as the following:
    ▪ thickening of the retina within 500 µm from the fovea
    ▪ hard exudates and adjacent thickening of the retina within 500 µm from the fovea
    ▪ area of retinal thickening one disc size (or larger), part of which is one disc diameter from the fovea.
  ○ To put these distances into perspective, the diameter of the disc is 1500 µm: so to assess CSMO, use one-third of this distance.
  ○ There are two main types of CSMO (ischaemic versus non-ischaemic): distinguishing is via fundus fluoroscein angiogram (FFA) and dictates management (Figure 45.6b).

Screening
• The screening service in the United Kingdom is a robust method of detecting early changes.
• Annual digital photographic screening in the community is mandatory for diabetic patients.
• Patients with at least R2 or M1 disease must be seen by an ophthalmologist (within 10 and 2 weeks, respectively).

KEY POINTS

• DR is the leading cause of blindness in the working population of the developed world.
• Screening and early treatment can prevent vision loss.
• Poorly controlled HbA1C and hypercholesterolaemia can accelerate DR changes.
• Rapid reduction in HbA1C over a short period of time can also accelerate DR changes.

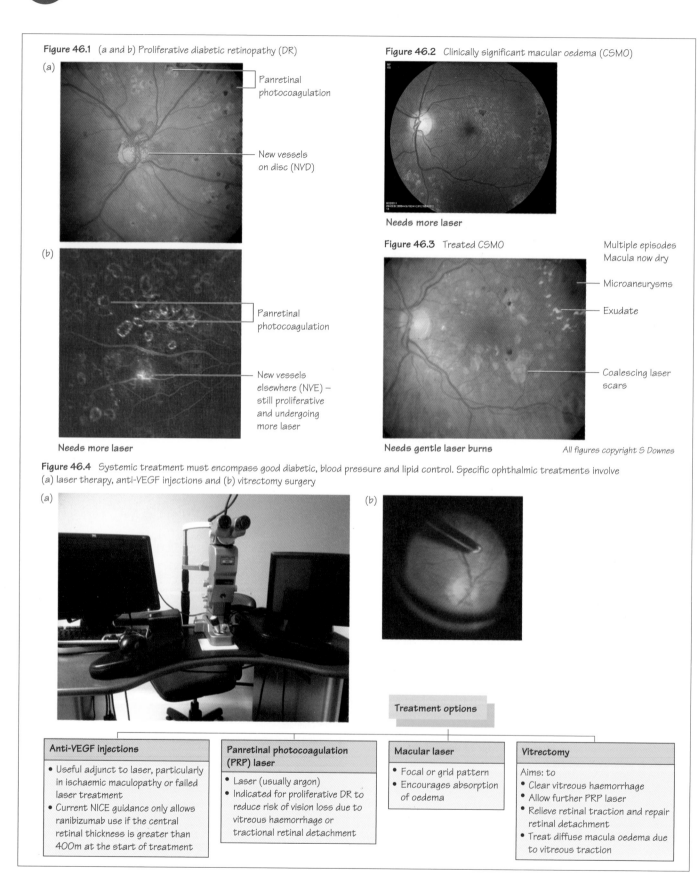

Figure 46.1 (a and b) Proliferative diabetic retinopathy (DR)

(a)

Panretinal photocoagulation

New vessels on disc (NVD)

(b)

Panretinal photocoagulation

New vessels elsewhere (NVE) – still proliferative and undergoing more laser

Needs more laser

Figure 46.2 Clinically significant macular oedema (CSMO)

Needs more laser

Figure 46.3 Treated CSMO

Multiple episodes Macula now dry

Microaneurysms

Exudate

Coalescing laser scars

Needs gentle laser burns

All figures copyright S Downes

Figure 46.4 Systemic treatment must encompass good diabetic, blood pressure and lipid control. Specific ophthalmic treatments involve (a) laser therapy, anti-VEGF injections and (b) vitrectomy surgery

(a)

(b)

Treatment options

Anti-VEGF injections
- Useful adjunct to laser, particularly in ischaemic maculopathy or failed laser treatment
- Current NICE guidance only allows ranibizumab use if the central retinal thickness is greater than 400m at the start of treatment

Panretinal photocoagulation (PRP) laser
- Laser (usually argon)
- Indicated for proliferative DR to reduce risk of vision loss due to vitreous haemorrhage or tractional retinal detachment

Macular laser
- Focal or grid pattern
- Encourages absorption of oedema

Vitrectomy

Aims: to
- Clear vitreous haemorrhage
- Allow further PRP laser
- Relieve retinal traction and repair retinal detachment
- Treat diffuse macula oedema due to vitreous traction

Ophthalmology at a Glance, Second Edition. Jane Olver, Lorraine Cassidy, Gurjeet Jutley, and Laura Crawley. © 2014 Jane Olver, Lorraine Cassidy, Gurjeet Jutley and Laura Crawley. Published 2014 by John Wiley & Sons, Ltd. Companion Website: www.ataglanceseries.com/ophthal

Aims

- Understand that systemic control is key in treatment.
- Appreciate the various management options in treating diabetic retinopathy.

Blood pressure (BP), lipid and glycaemic control

Control of these will:

- Reduce the progression and severity of diabetic retinopathy (DR): aim to bring down HbA1C slowly to 6.5–7.0%. If it comes down too quickly, there will be a transient worsening of the retinopathy.
- Reduce the need for laser treatment.

- Patients should also be advised not to smoke as this contributes to vascular damage.
- The Action to Control Cardiovascular Risk in Diabetes (ACCORD) study suggests that DR progression in type 2 diabetics is reduced by intensive glycaemic and lipid control, and only regular BP control.
- Patients benefit from the pleiotropic effects of statins and should be started on them even if lipid levels are in the normal range. It was shown in 2005 that these wider effects of statins include improving endothelial cell function, decreasing oxidative stress and inflammation and inhibiting the thrombogenic response.
- The Fenofibrate Intervention and Event Lowering in Diabetes (FIELD) study showed less progression to macular oedema and proliferative disease if patients were administered fenofibrate (the mechanism is more than just lipid lowering).

Treatment options

Prior to any laser, one must have a fundus flourescein angiography (FFA). This will give conclusive diagnosis of new vessels (which can be clinically difficult to distinguish from an intra-retinal microvascular abnormality). More importantly, it can differentiate ischaemic maculopathy (do **not** laser) from non-ischaemic (treat with laser).

Panretinal photocoagulation (PRP)

- Indicated for proliferative DR (Figure 46.1), rubeosis and vitreous haemorrhage (with adequate view).
- Laser photocoagulation is used to produce 1500–3000 burns of between 200 and 400 μm diameter in the peripheral retina, sparing the macula, papillomacular bundle and optic nerve head. This causes regression of neovascularization of the optic disc (NVD) and neovascularization elsewhere (NVE). The patient will have reduced peripheral and night vision post PRP. Transient worsening of central vision may be noted.
- PRP is performed in the outpatient clinic using a laser attached to a slit lamp. The treatment requires topical anaesthesia as a special contact lens is used to apply the laser burns. Once adequate laser has been applied, the abnormal vessels will regress in about 8 weeks.
- When counselling patients prior to the procedure, one should quote figures from the Early Treatment Diabetic Retinopathy Study (ETDRS) study. The risk of severe visual loss within 2 years in patients with high-risk proliferative DR reduces from 38% to 19% with PRP.

Macular laser (Figures 46.2 and 46.3a)

- This can be focal or grid, depending on whether a local or diffuse leakage pattern is seen.
- Patients must be warned that macular laser treatment is used to prevent vision from getting worse, but it does not always improve visual acuity. Some patients notice a scotoma after macular laser treatment.

- Again, patients can be informed of the data from the ETDRS study, which showed that the risk of moderate visual loss of three lines over 3 years was reduced from 24% to 12%.

Vitrectomy (Figure 46.3b)

This is a specialized procedure performed by a vitreo-retinal surgeon, whereby the vitreous is removed via a three-port pars plana incision (TPPV). The indications are:

- To clear vitreous haemorrhage—allowing the surgeon to visualize the retina and apply further PRP laser.
- To relieve retinal traction and repair retinal detachment.
- To treat diffuse macula oedema due to vitreous traction.

Clinical evidence for treatment

- The initial evidence for the use of macular laser was shown in the ETDRS study in 1985. However, only 3% of treated eyes actually have visual improvement, seen as letters gained on the LogMar chart.
- Rather, it is a measure to reduce the risk of visual loss in patients with clinically significant macular oedema (CSMO).
- Whilst laser will remain the gold standard treatment, recent advances include the administration of pharmacological agents into the vitreous cavity, such as steroidal and anti-VEGF (vascular endothelial growth factor) agents.
- These are now being used increasingly in clinical practice. A plethora of evidence supports the use of anti-VEGF agents, including four studies comparing intravenous (IV) ranibizumab with the gold standard (laser):
  - **DRCR.net:**
    - It was shown that ranibizumab with laser is more effective than laser alone after 1 year (gain of 9 letters versus 3, respectively).
  - **READ-2:**
    - At 6 months, patients gained more letters with ranibizumab alone, compared to in combination with laser or laser alone (7.2, 3.8 and 0.4, respectively).
  - **RESTORE:**
    - The same results as the READ-2 study were seen in the RESTORE study.
    - **And** the benefit was still evident after 12 months (a 6.1-letter gain in the ranibizumab monotherapy group, 5.9-letter gain in the ranibizumab and laser group and 0.8-letter gain in the laser-only group).
  - **RESOLVE:**
    - Ranibizumab was superior to sham injections, with patients gaining 10.3 letters at 12 months (compared to −1.4 letters with sham and rescue laser).

- Hence, over the next few years we will see the use of IV agents and combination therapy used readily to treat CSMO.
- The upcoming RIDE and RISE studies will give more indication as to whether injections should be given in a monthly fashion, regardless of clinical response, or on a *pro re nata* basis.

KEY POINTS

- Tight BP, lipid and glycaemic control reduces the progression and severity of DR and must be emphasized to patients **regardless** of any ocular therapy.
- PRP is the treatment for proliferative DR.
- Focal laser, intra-vitreal therapy and a combination of the two are used to treat leaking microaneurysms at the macula that are threatening vision.

Anatomy

Figure 47.1 Central retinal artery course at the optic nerve head

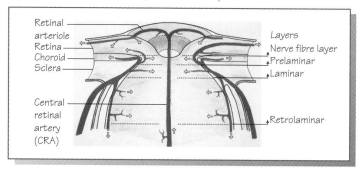

Retinal arteriole
Retina
Choroid
Sclera

Central retinal artery (CRA)

Layers
Nerve fibre layer
Prelaminar
Laminar
Retrolaminar

Figure 47.2 Human methylmethacrylate vascular cast with a view of posterior cerebral artery supply to the choroids and retrolaminar optic nerve

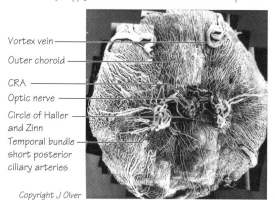

Vortex vein
Outer choroid
CRA
Optic nerve
Circle of Haller and Zinn
Temporal bundle short posterior ciliary arteries

Copyright J Olver

Figure 47.3 Choroid with retinal arteriole and residual capillaries

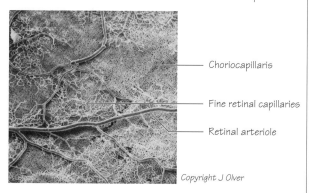

Choriocapillaris
Fine retinal capillaries
Retinal arteriole

Copyright J Olver

All tissue has been dissolved away from the intralumen vascular casts

Figure 47.4 Central retinal artery occlusion (CRAO) causing (a) a cherry red spot and (b) a very ischaemic retina

(a)

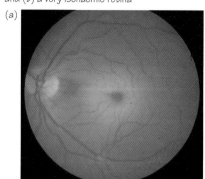

(b)

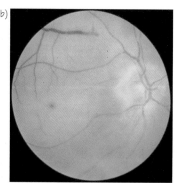

Figure 47.5 Inferior hemi-retinal artery occlusion

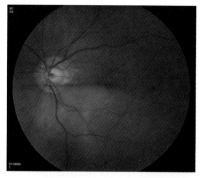

Figure 47.6 CRAO with cilioretinal sparing. A central patch of vision is maintained

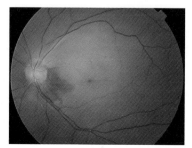

Figure 47.7 Branch retinal artery occlusion. The arrow points to the occluded branch

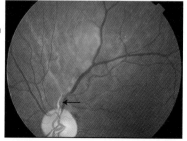

You should recognize sudden painless loss of vision from a central retinal artery occlusion (CRAO). It is an ocular emergency (see also Chapter 20).

Aims
- Understand the vascular anatomy of the retina and optic nerve head.
- Identify the clinical features of a CRAO.
- Be able to manage a patient with CRAO.

Anatomy (Figures 47.1, 47.2 and 47.3)
The eye has a rich blood supply from the ophthalmic artery via the central retinal artery (CRA) and the posterior ciliary arteries (PCAs). The CRA supplies the superficial nerve fibre layer and inner two-thirds of the retina. The PCAs supply the rest of the anterior optic nerve and uvea (iris, ciliary body and choroid), and hence the deep retinal layers. The anatomy is known from vascular casts (in vitro) and from live fluorescein angiographic studies. In vascular casts of the eye, the cadaver ophthalmic artery has been injected with a plastic and the tissue has dissolved away, leaving only the vessel lumen—the cast.

The CRA is an end artery of the ophthalmic artery, which supplies the inner two-thirds of the retina. The choriocapillaris, supplied by the posterior ciliary arteries, supplies the outer retina.

> **WARNING**
>
> ▶ CRA obstruction causes ischaemia of the inner retinal layers, resulting in oedema of the nerve fibre layer (NFL) (Figure 47.4).

Urgent

If blood flow is not restored within 100 min, irreversible damage occurs at its narrowest point, which is the lamina cribrosa. A blockage more distally gives rise to a branch artery occlusion. Central retinal or hemiretinal artery occlusions (Figure 48.5) are more common than a branch retinal arteriole occlusion (Figure 47.6).

Pathology

Arterial occlusion results from	Inner retinal ischaemia causes	Retinal infarction gives rise to
• Circulating embolus (e.g. heart or carotids) • Local atheroma • Arteritis (e.g. giant cell arteritis) • Miscellaneous (e.g. migraine, syphilis and herpes zoster)	• Intracellular oedema—the retina appears white, which masks the choroidal circulation, except at the macula 'cherry red spot'.	• Loss of NFL • Pale optic disc

Cilioretinal artery
Note that 15–20% of individuals have a supplementary arterial supply to the macula via a cilioretinal artery derived from the posterior ciliary circulation at the disc. In the event of a CRAO, the macula would remain perfused in these patients with some preservation of vision (Figure 47.7).

Diagnosis and management
Symptoms
- Painless loss of vision (note that non-ocular pain may occur such as temporal or scalp tenderness in giant cell arteritis (GCA)).
- Profound drop in visual acuity (unless cilioretinal artery sparing).
- Afferent papillary defect.

Signs
Perform a dilated fundal examination to detect:
- cherry red spot at the macula (Figure 47.4a)
- embolus occasionally visible at the optic disc
- attenuation of arterioles
- retinal pallor
- mild disc swelling.

Treatment
The aim is to re-establish circulation within the CRA. This is attempted by:
- Lowering the intraocular pressure (IOP) using:
  - acetazolamide 500 mg IV
  - ocular massage
  - anterior chamber paracentesis (1 ml aqueous withdrawn).
- Vasodilation: rebreathe into a paper bag (carbon dioxide increases).
- Start cholesterol-lowering statins (e.g. Simvastatin and Atorvastatin).
- Start antiplatelets (e.g. aspirin 300 mg stat, then 75 mg daily or clopidogrel 75 mg daily) within 48 hr.

> **WARNING**
>
> ▶ It is *essential* to check the erythrocyte sedimentation rate (ESR) and C-reactive protein to investigate for an inflammatory cause for CRAO, since GCA is often a bilateral condition with catastrophic visual loss if not treated appropriately.

Outcome
Visual recovery is dependent on the interval between onset and presentation. There has not been a clinical trial comparing treatment versus no treatment—but it is believed that 66% of patients have vision <6/60 following CRAO.

Other investigations
Examine for carotid bruits, heart murmurs and irregular pulse (atrial fibrillation is a cause—needs anticoagulation). Arrange carotid Doppler studies, 24 h Holter monitor and echocardiogram. Follow-up is by a physician.

> **KEY POINTS**
>
> - The CRA supplies the inner two-thirds of the retina.
> - Check the ESR in all cases of CRAO to exclude GCA.
> - A cilioretinal artery is present in 15–20% of individuals, which affords some protection from severe visual loss.

The central retinal vein drains all the layers of the retina and the optic nerve head anterior to the lamina cribosa. When it is occluded, there is marked venous engorgement and leakage with retinal oedema, ischaemia and haemorrhage

Figure 48.1 Anatomy of the central retinal vein (CRV) course at the optic nerve head

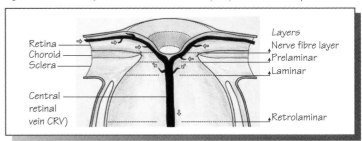

Retina
Choroid
Sclera

Central retinal vein CRV)

Layers
Nerve fibre layer
Prelaminar
Laminar
Retrolaminar

Figure 48.2 Human methylmethacrylate vascular casts. (a) The optic disc: retinal venule tributaries form the central retinal vein deep in the optic cup and (b) an isolated retinal cast with the central retinal artery and vein

All tissue has been dissolved away from the intralumen vascular casts

(a)

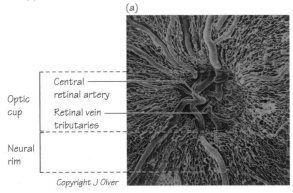

Optic cup

Central retinal artery
Retinal vein tributaries

Neural rim

Copyright J Olver

(b)

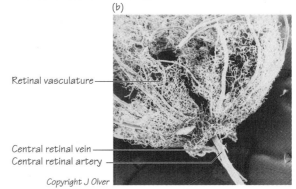

Retinal vasculature

Central retinal vein
Central retinal artery

Copyright J Olver

Figure 48.3 Central retinal vein occlusion (CRVO) (left eye)

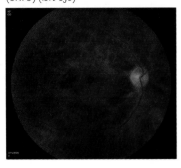

Figure 48.4 Neovascular glaucoma – iris new vessels and pathology.
(a) Rubeosis iridis (iris neovascularization) – end-stage disease; and
(b) histopathology of iris surface with arrows showing iris neovascularization

(a)   (b)

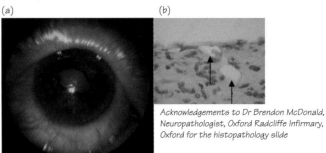

Acknowledgements to Dr Brendon McDonald, Neuropathologist, Oxford Radcliffe Infirmary, Oxford for the histopathology slide

Figure 48.6 Superior hemi-retinal vein occlusion

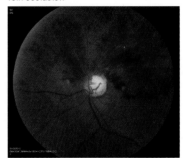

Figure 48.5 Branch retinal vein occlusion (BRVO) affecting (a) three quadrants (left eye) and (b) one quadrant (right eye). (c) A fluorescein angiogram of branch vein occlusion

(a)   (b)   (c)

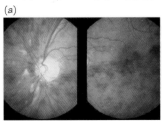 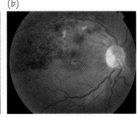 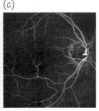

Table 48.1 Risk factors for vein occlusion, in order of decreasing association

All must be considered once diagnosis is made:
- Hypertension
- Diabetes mellitus
- Hyperlipidaemia
- Smoking
- Glaucoma
- Thrombophilia and Inflammatory conditions

For other causes of painless loss of vision, see Chapter 20.

Aims
- Identify the clinical features of central and branch retinal vein occlusion.
- Updates on managing vein occlusions.

Retinal vein occlusion
This is a common cause of painless loss of vision. It can occur at any age, with 85% of patients aged >50 years. It's classified into central retinal vein occlusion (CRVO), branch retinal vein occlusion (BRVO) and hemispheric retinal vein occlusion (HRVO), depending on the site of the obstruction. See Table 48.1 for associated risk factors.

Pathology of visual loss in vein occlusion
- Macular oedema:
  ○ caused predominantly by increased venous pressure (intraluminal), vasoactive / inflammatory mediators (such as vascular endothelial growth factor [VEGF]) and dysregulation of tight junctions
- Ischaemia:
  ○ this can be isolated (macular ischaemia) or generalized retinal ischaemia.
  ○ Significant generalised retinal ischaemia can lead to ocular neovascularization via hypoxia induced production of vasoactive mediators, with VEGF being the primary mediator (neovascularization in the anterior segment (iris new vessels) results in rubeotic glaucoma; neovascularization in the posterior segment (new vessels on the disc and new vessels elsewhere) can result in vitreous haemorrhage and tractional retinal detachment.

Visual prognosis and management depend on the type of occlusion, the severity of the occlusion and the ocular sequelae. Visual loss is worse in CRVO than BRVO/HRVO. Some small BRVOs are asymptomatic, especially if they are located in only one quadrant nasal to the disc (i.e. away from the macula).

Central retinal vein occlusion
The central retinal vein (CRV) (Figures 48.1 and 48.2) deep in the optic cup is occluded, affecting drainage from all four retinal quadrants, resulting in usually unilateral painless visual loss (Figure 48.3). The pathogenesis of CRVO is believed to be due to in situ thrombosis in the CRV.

Ischaemic CRVO
25 to 33% of cases are ischaemic, associated with new vessel formation on the iris (rubeosis iridis), disc or elsewhere (Figure 48.4). Ultimately these vessels can result in visual loss, either by occluding and contracting the irido-corneal angle (rubeotic glaucoma) or by bleeding (vitreous haemorrhage) and exerting traction on the retina.

Ischaemic CRVO requires panretinal photocoagulation (PRP) laser treatment to reduce the aforementioned risk of visual loss.

Signs include:
- relative afferent pupillary defect (RAPD) and markedly reduced vision (often 6/60 or less)
- extensive widespread deep retinal haemorrhages
- multiple widespread cotton wool spots
- large areas of capillary non-perfusion (detected with FFA).

Non-ischaemic CRVO
- Variable number of haemorrhages in 4 quadrants
- Tortuous dilated retinal veins
- No RAPD and visual loss not as profound as in ischaemic CRVO (usually better than 6/60)
- Neovascularization of anterior or posterior segment is rare in true non-ischaemic CRVO (<2% incidence)
- 30% of cases convert to the ischaemic form, and usually associated with further visual deterioration
- Recovery to normal vision is seen in fewer than 10% of cases.

Branch retinal vein occlusion (Figure 48.5)
BRVOs are three times more common than CRVOs and occur at arteriovenous crossings where the artery and vein share a common advential sheath. It is postulated that the rigid artery compresses the retinal vein, which results in turbulent flow and endothelial damage, followed by thrombosis and obstruction of the retinal vein. Patients present with painless loss of central vision, or as an incidental finding if the macula is not involved. Retinal haemorrhages and cotton wool spots are confined to one area. BRVO is superotemporal in more than 60% of cases, suggested to be due to the increased number of arteriovenous crossings in that quadrant. BRVO can be ischaemic or non-ischaemic. Hypertension is the most common association of BRVO. Macular oedema and retinal/disc neovascularization are the major complications requiring intervention, with rubeosis much less common compared with CRVO.

Usually, the central retinal vein is formed ahead of the opening in the sclera and leaves the eye with the artery, to drain directly into the cavernous sinus or superior ophthalmic vein. However, in 20% of the population, two branch retinal veins, draining the superior and inferior halves of the retina respectively, leave the eye. Hence, the central retinal vein forms posterior to the scleral opening (i.e. the lamina cribrosa). A hemispheric vein occlusion is an occlusion of one of these trunks (Figure 48.6). They can also be either ischaemic or non-ischaemic. They are often managed as per a BRVO.

Management
Medical management
- Check blood pressure, full blood count (FBC), erythrocyte sedimentation rate (ESR), urea and electrolytes (U&E), lipid profile, blood sugar, and plasma proteins.
- In a young patient, a thrombophilia screen must be done, including:
  ○ protein C
  ○ protein S
  ○ anti-cardiolipin Ab
  ○ anti-nuclear Ab
  ○ factor V Leiden's mutation.
  ○ plasma homocysteine
- Medical treatment of cardiovascular risk factors
- Aspirin
- Treat raised intraocular pressure (IOP).

Current treatment (Detailed guidelines can be found on the Royal College website)

Ischaemic CRVO

• Monthly follow-up.

• PRP is required with onset of new vessels (anterior or posterior segment).

• Consider adjunctive intravitreal anti-VEGF agents, including bevacizumab, to help manage iris new vessels in the acute phase.

Rubeotic glaucoma (typically occurs at 3 months, hence '100-day glaucoma')

• If no visual potential = atropine and steroids.

• If visual potential = Following complete PRP—IOP control, cyclo-ablation and/or surgery to lower IOP.

Macular oedema secondary to non-ischaemic BRVO and non-ischaemic CRVO

• Intravitreal therapies are being increasingly employed for macular oedema without significantly compromised macular perfusion—including a biodegradable dexamethasone implant (Ozurdex), and intravitreal ranibizumab / bevacizumab / aflibercept.

• Macular photocoagulation can still be considered in patients with BRVO and vision 6/12 or worse, and more than 3 month duration of macular oedema.

Important studies

Branch vein occlusion study (BVOS)

• Landmark study as it was the first to advocate treatment of macular oedema based on a randomized controlled trial.

• Twice as many patients treated with laser, compared to the control group, gained two lines at 3 years.

• Evidence from this trial established macular laser as the gold standard treatment for 25 years.

• It also demonstrated that scatter laser photocoagulation could significantly prevent the development of both neovascularization and vitreous haemorrhage. The data suggested that peripheral scatter laser be applied after, rather than before, the development of neovascularization.

Central retinal vein occlusion study (CVOS)

• Showed that macular laser did not improve vision for patients with oedema secondary to CRVO.

• Prophylactic PRP did not prevent the development of rubeosis. This suggested that with careful follow-up it is safe to wait for the development of early iris neovascularization and then apply PRP.

Standard care vs. corticosteroid for retinal vein occlusion (SCORE)—BRVO

• Twenty-five years on from BVOS, the first trial to compare a treatment against the gold standard of macular laser.

• Intravitreal triamcinolone (Trivaris) has **no** benefit over laser in patients with BRVO.

• The effect is transient and repeat injections may be necessary. Also, the risk of glaucoma and cataract development is significant.

Standard care vs. corticosteroid for retinal vein occlusion (SCORE)—CRVO

• Intravitreal triamcinolone was found to be superior to observation for treating vision loss associated with macular edema secondary to non-ischaemic CRVO.

• The 1 mg dose has a safety profile superior to that of the 4 mg dose.

• As with SCORE BRVO repeat injections are likely to be necessary, with significant risk of glaucoma and cataract development.

GENEVA

• Patients with macular oedema from either CRVO or BRVO were given either a dexamethasone implant or sham.

• The implant is approved by NICE for non-ischaemic CRVO and indicated in BRVO if laser treatment has not been beneficial, or is not possible due to the extent of macular haemorrhage.

• Regular monitoring of IOP required. Moderate IOP rise in 15%, peaking at 2 months following implant. Cataract formation often accelerated.

BRAVO

• Patients with macular oedema secondary to BRVO were randomized to sham, 0.5 mg or 0.3 mg ranibizumab.

• At 12 months, the mean letter gains were 12.1, 18.3 and 16.6, respectively.

• Treatment has now been approved by NICE.

CRUISE

• Patients with macular oedema secondary to non-ischaemic CRVO were randomized to sham, 0.5 mg or 0.3 mg ranibizumab.

• At 12 months, the mean letter gains were 7.3, 14.9 and 12.7, respectively.

• Treatment has now been approved by NICE.

KEY POINTS

• Retinal Vein Occlusions are common causes of painless visual loss and are primarily a result of atherosclerosis.

• RVOs can be either ischaemic or non-ischaemic—with neovascularization secondary to ischaemia managed by PRP.

• Macular Oedema is a common complication that is increasingly being managed by intravitreal therapies.

Eyelids

Figure 49.1 (a) *Molluscum contagiosum* on eyelid (usually multiple in HIV), (b) kaposi sarcoma lower eyelid and (c) herpes zoster ophthalmicus (i) plus maxillary branch involvement (ii)

(a)

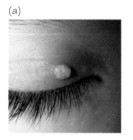

(b)

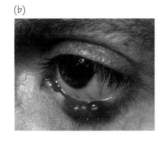

(c) (i)

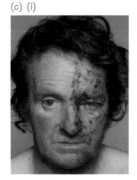

(ii)

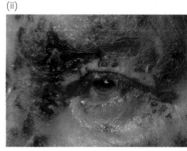

Figure 49.2 Retinal ischaemia showing cotton wool spots

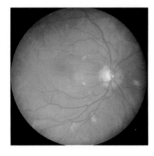

Retinal/choroidal infections

Figure 49.3 Cytomegalovirus (CMV) (a) papillitis and (b) chorioretinitis

(a)

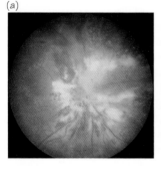

(b)

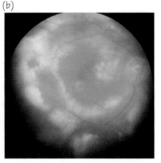

Figure 49.4 Toxoplasmosis retinochoroiditis

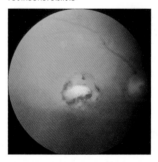

Figure 49.5 Syphilis can manifest anywhere in the eye. This photo shows choroiditis and optic nerve oedema

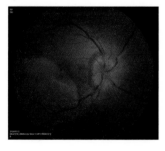

Figure 49.6 Varicella zoster virus retinitis (VZVR)

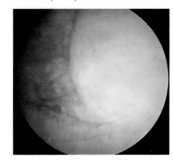

Figure 49.7 *Pneumocystis carinii* pneumonia (PCP) choroiditis

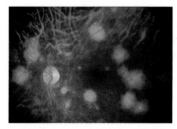

VZVR, CMV, toxoplasmosis retinochoroiditis and candida endophthalmitis may cause severe visual loss. PCP and cryptococcal retinitis is treatable

With current antiretrovirals, there is less advanced HIV ocular involvement. Be alert to a diagnosis of HIV in adults with unexplained eyelid, orbital and retinal disease.

Aims

Know how:
• HIV-related disease affects the eye and can lead to permanent visual loss.
• Treatment of specific ophthalmic opportunistic infections.

HIV modes of transmission

• Sexual transmission (homosexual and heterosexual)
• Parenteral transmission with blood and blood products: semen from artificial insemination and organ transplantation
• Occupational risk: small risk for healthcare workers of 0.3% after a single percutaneous exposure to HIV-infected blood. Infection risk also from blood contamination of mucous membranes, non-intact skin and conjunctiva
• Perinatal transmission: accounts for 80–90% of all paediatric HIV infections. Congenital HIV infection may occur transplacentally or intrapartum. The majority of infection occurs during birth or from breastfeeding
• Other routes: no evidence of HIV transmission from tears, sweat, urine or other body fluids
• NB. 30–50% of the non-HIV population will have serological evidence of previous toxoplasmosis

Ophthalmologic disorders in HIV

Patients with HIV/AIDS who have CD4 counts less than 50 per µl are at high risk of developing opportunistic infections in the eye.

Ophthalmic problems in AIDS can involve any ocular or orbital tissue, but the sight-threatening disease affects the posterior segment. The incidence of posterior infections is much less frequent since the advent of highly active antiretroviral therapy (HAART). Note that there is **no** evidence that HIV can be transmitted via tears, and no extra precaution need be taken when examining patients in clinic.

The following occur in various parts of the eye in those with low CD4 counts:

Adnexa and anterior segment (Figure 49.1)
• Molluscum contagiosum on eyelids (Figure 49.1a)
• HIV-related conjunctivitis
• Kaposi's sarcoma—flat or raised (if present >4/12) violaceous vascular conjunctival lesion, surrounded by tortuous and dilated vessels (Figure 49.1b). Treated by excision, chemotherapy or radiotherapy.

• Conjunctival granulomas due to cryptococcal infection, tuberculosis and other mycotic infections
• Aggressive conjunctival or cutaneous eyelid squamous cell carcinoma (see Chapter 26). Associated with human papillomavirus infection.
• Herpes zoster ophthalmicus (HZO): also often affects the seventh cranial nerve (Figure 49.1c).
• Herpes simplex keratitis
• Microsporidia: a protozoal infection causing coarse, superficial, punctate keratitis with minimal conjunctival reaction.

Orbit
• Periorbital B cell lymphoma
• Burkitt's lymphoma
• Kaposi's sarcoma.

Posterior segment

HIV retinopathy (microvascular disease) (Figure 49.2)
• Comprises cotton wool spots, retinal haemorrhages, microaneurysms and ischaemic maculopathy.

Immune recovery uveitis (IRU)
• Occurs in eye with quiescent cytomegalovirus retinitis (CMVR) in patients responding to HAART, defined as vitritis of ≥1+ *or* trace of cells plus epiretinal membrane *or* cystoid macular oedema.

Retinal opportunistic infections
• CMVR (Figure 49.3)
  ○ 'Pizza pie fundus': haemorrhagic or non-haemorrhagic, frosted-branch angiitis or mimics central retinal vein occlusion.
• Toxoplasmosis retinochoroiditis (*Toxoplasma gondii*) (Figure 49.4)
  ○ White or yellow patch of focal retinal necrosis
  ○ In the immunocompromised, lesions tend to be larger; bilateral disease in 18–38%; unusual forms occur (solitary, multifocal or miliary), minimal vitritis; prolonged therapy is required.
• Syphilitic retinitis (Figure 49.5)
  ○ Syphilis is the great mimic and can present as vitritis, multifocal choroiditis, retinal vasculitis, neuroretinitis, optic atrophy or oedema, exudative retinal detachment, choroidal effusion, pigmentary retinopathy and venous and arterial occlusions.
• Cryptococcal choroiditis (*Cryptococcus neoformans*)
  ○ Variably sized deep choroidal infiltrates; may be asymptomatic.
• Mycobacterium tuberculosis choroiditis
  ○ Single large granuloma or multifocal; plus or minus retinal vasculitis; frequently bilateral; choroidal neovascularization may develop at sites of healed spots.
• Candida endophthalmitis (*Candida albicans*)
  ○ Small, whitish, multifocal, circumscribed chorioretinal infiltrates; retinal haemorrhages; dense vitritis and 'fluff balls' (vitreous abscesses) progress to endophthalmitis
• Progressive outer retinal necrosis (PORN)
  ○ Herpes simplex virus or varicella zoster virus (Figure 49.6)
  ○ Multifocal deep retinal patches, predominantly at the posterior pole.
  ○ PORN affects the choroid, leading to round yellow-white flat lesions in the posterior pole (Figure 49.7). Visual symptoms are rarely seen.
• *Pneumocystis jirovecii*, formerly known as *P. carinii*
  ○ Pneumocystis pneumonia (PCP) is caused by a yeast-like fungus. Predominantly affects the lungs.

Primary intraocular B cell lymphoma
• Typically high grade; significant vitritis with or without iritis; peri-papillary infiltrates; disc swelling; yellow-white sub-RPE lesions; vascular sheathing and vein or artery occlusion.

WARNING

▶ Varicella zoster virus retinitis (VZVR)—may blind patients.
▶ Acute retinal necrosis (ARN) occurs in the immunocompetent, whereas PORN occurs in the immunosuppressed.
▶ PORN: bilateral multifocal retinitis with opacification in the outer retina and rapid progression. Minimal or no vitritis. Very poor prognosis with standard therapies, leading to blindness in most cases.

Visual prognosis

• VZVR, CMVR, toxoplasmosis retinochoroiditis and candida endophthalmitis may cause severe visual loss.
• PCP and cryptococcal retinitis are treatable

Neuro-ophthalmic disorders in HIV

• You must always assess for a relative afferent pupillary defect in HIV patients as quite often the optic disc is involved:
  ◦ Optic disc swelling secondary to cryptococcal meningitis.
  ◦ Optic atrophy secondary to retinal disease.
• Look carefully for bilateral swollen optic discs, as papilloedema can be evident secondary to:
  ◦ Progressive multifocal leucoencephalopathy (PML)
  ◦ Cerebral infarction
  ◦ Intracranial toxoplasmosis
  ◦ Lymphoma.
• Cranial nerve palsies can be secondary to intracranial space-occupying lesions or infection.

Treatment
Ophthalmologists liaise with HIV physicians to ensure that patients are controlled on triple or quadruple HAART treatments.
• CMVR
  ◦ Various regimes include:
    ▪ Oral valganciclovir
    ▪ Intravenous gancyclovir
    ▪ Sustained-release gancyclovir implanted directly into the vitreous. A trial in 1997 showed that an implant reduces the risk of progressive retinitis by one-third in comparison with intravenous gancyclovir. Each implant lasts for 5–8 months; it needs to be replaced surgically.
• Toxoplasmosis
  ◦ Treatment with clindamycin, pyrimethamine, azithromycin and atovoquone.
  ◦ **No** place for steroids in toxoplasma infection in the immunocompromised.

KEY POINTS

• HZO or multiple molluscum contagiosum in a young adult may indicate HIV.
• Opportunistic infections are on the decline due to HAART.

---

50 Tropical ophthalmology: tropical eye disease

Figure 50.1 Summary of the Trachoma Grading System: (a) trachomatous trichiasis (TT), (b) corneal opacity (CO), (c) a normal, healthy eye without inflammation, where the eyelid has been everted, (d) trachomatous inflammation—follicular (TF), (e) trachomatous inflammation—intense (TI) and (f) trachomatous scarring (TS).
Photos by Murray McGavin, Hugh Taylor and John DC Anderson. Images courtesy of International Centre for Eye Health Image Library.

(a) (b) (c)

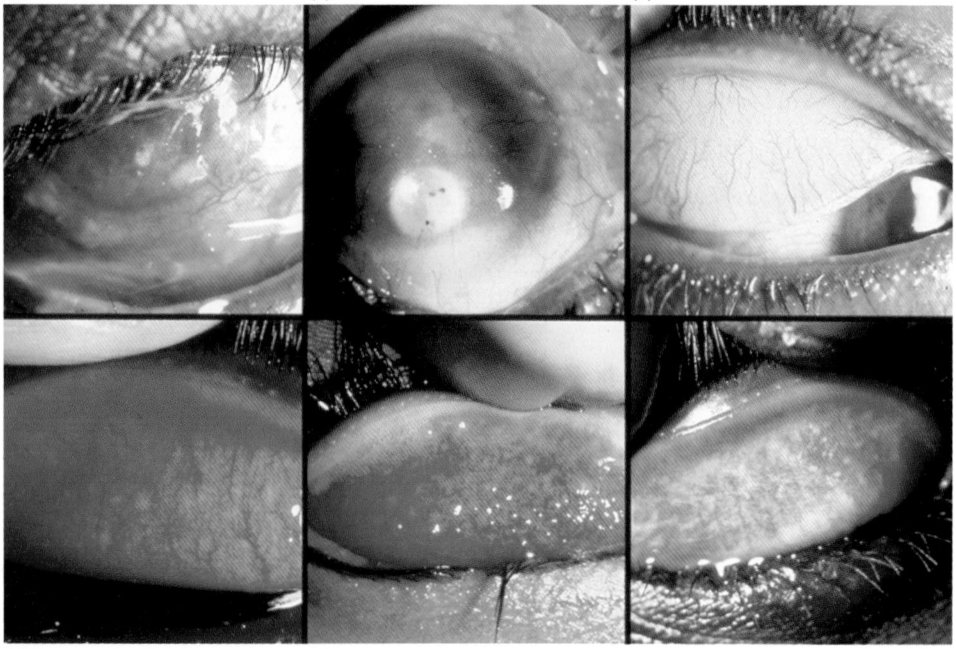

(d) (e) (f)

Figure 50.2 Skin disease in onchocerciasis
Image courtesy of International Centre for Eye Health Image Library

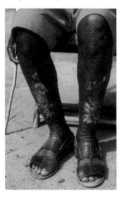

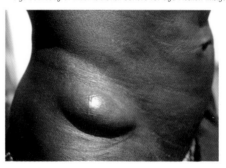

Figure 50.4 Sclerosing keratitis from onchocerciasis.
Image courtesy of International Centre for Eye Health Image Library

Figure 50.3 Onchocerciasis nodule on bony prominence.
Image courtesy of International Centre for Eye Health Image Library

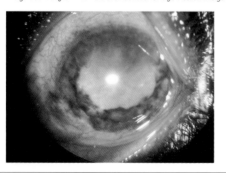

Figure 50.5 Eye of a small girl with acute keratomalacia: the cornea has almost completely melted away, with no inflammatory reaction. *Photo by Margreet Hogeweg. Image courtesy of International Centre for Eye Health Image Library*

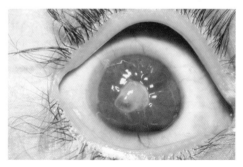

Aims

• Epidemiology of tropical eye disease.
• Understand how the causes of blindness and low vision vary globally.

These conditions are not commonly seen in the United Kingdom. You may come across them if you undertake a medical elective in a tropical country, or if a patient comes from a country where the disease is endemic. They are important causes of global blindness.

Trachoma

• Caused by *Chlamydia trachomatis*—a microorganism that spreads through contact with eye discharge from the infected person (on towels, handkerchiefs, fingers etc.) and through transmission by eye-seeking flies.
• After years of repeated infection, the inside of the eyelid may be scarred so severely that the eyelid turns inwards (trichiasis) and the lashes rub on the eyeball, scarring the cornea. If untreated, this leads to the formation of irreversible corneal opacities and blindness (Figure 50.1).
• Affects about 84 million people, of whom about 8 million are visually impaired.
• Seen in many of the poorest and poor rural areas of Africa, Asia, Central and South America, Australia and the Middle East.
• Environmental risk factors are water shortage, flies, poor hygiene conditions and crowded households.
• Management is via the SAFE strategy. This consists of lid surgery (S), antibiotics to treat the community pool of infection (A), facial cleanliness (F) and environmental changes (E).

Onchocerciasis

• An insect-borne disease caused by a parasite, *Onchocerca volvulus*, and transmitted by blackflies of the species *Simulium damnosum*. Often called 'river blindness' because the blackfly that transmits the disease resides in fertile riverside areas.
• Adult worms of *O. volvulus* live in nodules in a human body, where the female worms produce high numbers of first-stage larvae known as microfilariae. They migrate from the nodules to the sub-epidermal layer of the skin, where they can be ingested by blackflies. They further develop in the body of the insect, from which more people can be infected (Figures 50.2, 50.3 and 50.4).
• Eye lesions in humans are caused by microfilariae. They can be found in all internal tissues of the eye where they cause inflammation, bleeding and other complications that can ultimately lead to blindness.

• This is a major cause of blindness in many African countries. It is also prevalent in Yemen and in Latin America. It is estimated that there are about half a million blind people due to river blindness.
• The disease can now also be treated with an annual dose of the drug ivermectin (Mectizan®), which also relieves the severe skin itching caused by the disease.

Leprosy

• Leprosy is caused by *Mycobacterium leprae*—predominantly seen in South America, South-east Asia and Africa.
• Leprosy is still endemic in many developing countries. It is estimated that 200 000–300 000 patients suffer from blindness.
• With modern anti-leprosy treatment, patients are made non-infectious almost immediately. Patients are generally treated as outpatients. Most people have a natural immunity against leprosy. Health workers who work with leprosy patients are unlikely to contract leprosy.
• Causes of blindness include iritis, exposure keratitis, corneal opacity, interstitial keratitis, chronic uveitis, cataract, glaucoma and trichiasis with corneal scarring.

Vitamin A deficiency (VAD) and measles

• Vitamin A in small amounts is necessary for the normal functioning of the visual system, erythropoiesis and immunity and to maintain cell growth and functioning.
• If a person eats an inadequate diet during critical stages of development, Vitamin A liver stores deplete and serum retinol concentrations become deficient, raising the risk of xerophthalmia.
• Xerophthalmia, which is caused by vitamin A deficiency and sometimes precipitated by measles, accounts for more than half of the new cases of childhood blindness each year. The conjunctiva becomes dry, thick and wrinkled. If untreated, it can lead to corneal ulceration and ultimately in blindness as a result of corneal damage (Figure 50.5).
• In addition to blindness, these young children are at increased risk of death. Prevention plays an important role: vitamin A supplementation, measles vaccination and nutritional advice have led to a marked reduction in this condition.

KEY POINTS

• Trachoma continues to be hyperendemic in many of the poorest parts of the world.
• Several of these conditions cause corneal scarring witch ultimately leads to functional vision loss.
• These conditions are related to poverty; improvement of sanitation and living conditions can reduce the incidence of these conditions.

Figure 51.1 Proportion of cases of blindness worldwide due to each major cause
Reproduced with permission from Foster A, Gilbert C, Johnson G. Changing patterns in global blindness: 1988–2008. Community Eye Health Journal. 2008;21:37–39
Global numbers shown in millions (m)

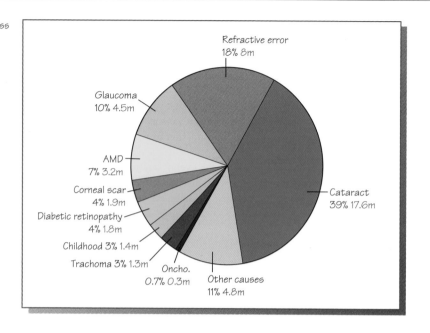

Refractive error 18% 8m

Glaucoma 10% 4.5m

AMD 7% 3.2m

Corneal scar 4% 1.9m

Diabetic retinopathy 4% 1.8m

Childhood 3% 1.4m

Trachoma 3% 1.3m

Oncho. 0.7% 0.3m

Other causes 11% 4.8m

Cataract 39% 17.6m

Figure 51.2 (a) Global causes of visual impairment, inclusive of blindness, as percentage of global visual impairment in 2010.
(b) Global causes of blindness as a percentage of global blindness in 2010.
AMD: Age-related macular degeneration; CO: corneal opacities; DR: diabetic retinopathy; RE: uncorrected refractive errors.
Reproduced from Pascolini D and Mariotti SP (2012). Global estimates of visual impairment: 2010. British Journal of Ophthalmology 96(5):614–618, with permission from BMJ Publishing Group Ltd

(a)

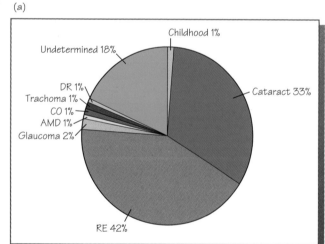

Childhood 1%
Undetermined 18%
DR 1%
Trachoma 1%
CO 1%
AMD 1%
Glaucoma 2%
Cataract 33%
RE 42%

(b)

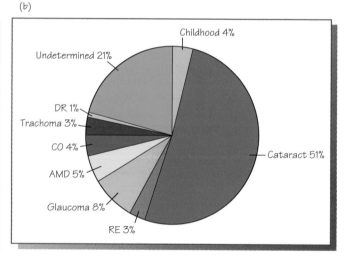

Childhood 4%
Undetermined 21%
DR 1%
Trachoma 3%
CO 4%
AMD 5%
Glaucoma 8%
RE 3%
Cataract 51%

Ophthalmology at a Glance, Second Edition. Jane Olver, Lorraine Cassidy, Gurjeet Jutley, and Laura Crawley. © 2014 Jane Olver, Lorraine Cassidy, Gurjeet Jutley and Laura Crawley. Published 2014 by John Wiley & Sons, Ltd. Companion Website: www.ataglanceseries.com/ophthal

Aims

- Epidemiology of tropical eye disease.
- Understand how the causes of blindness and low vision vary globally.

Introduction

Global estimates suggest that 285 million people are visually impaired worldwide, of which 39 million are blind and 246 have low vision (Figures 51.1 and 51.2). The number of people affected by infectious causes (e.g. trachoma, onchocerciasis and leprosy) has decreased over the last 20 years as access to improved diet, sanitation and antibiotics has increased. Almost 90% of blind people live in low-income countries.

Cataract (see Chapters 36–38)

Cataract is the leading cause of blindness worldwide. Seventeen million people globally are estimated to be blind from cataract. In well-resourced countries, cataract extraction by phacoemulsification is readily available. The introduction of a technique called small incision cataract surgery (SICS) has reduced the cost of surgery in low-income settings and has a faster recovery time. The availability of low-cost, good-quality intraocular lenses (IOLs) has increased the number of cataract surgeries and improved the visual outcome for patients. In some countries (e.g. Nigeria) couching is still practised, a procedure where a curved needle is used to dislocate the lens to the back of the eye. This leads to chronic ocular inflammation and poor vision.

Refractive error (see Chapters 8 and 9)

The World Health Organization definitions of blindness prior to 2008 failed to include correctable refractive error; it has only recently been recognized as a cause of avoidable blindness. It is estimated that 43% of global visual impairment is due to uncorrected refractive errors. Spectacles that are low cost and good quality are becoming more available, but in many countries there is still a need for good refraction services and optometrists.

Glaucoma (see Chapters 39–41)

Due to the lack of a proper definition or to the constant revision of the definition and classification of glaucoma, the estimated number of individuals blinded by this condition might be falsely low. It has been suggested that 60 million people are likely to have some form of glaucoma, and 8 million are likely to be blind. In many low- and middle-income countries, effective treatment for glaucoma is inaccessible. Medical treatment requires the availability of affordable drugs and long-term follow-up. Surgical treatment requires skilled surgical expertise and experience; patient acceptance is also a factor—in some African countries, the word for 'surgery' is the same word used for butchery of animals.

Age-related Macular Degeneration (AMD)

(see Chapter 44)

AMD is responsible for 7% of all blindness worldwide, ranging from close to 0% in sub-Saharan Africa to 50% in industrialized countries.

With an aging population, the number of AMD cases is likely to increase globally. The number affected is expected to double by the year 2020. The main risk factors are age, race, smoking, a family history of the condition, hypertension, high cholesterol, high fat intake and high Body Mass Index. The complement factor H gene has also been implicated. Current available treatments are expensive, and low-vision aids can also be difficult to access in resource-limited settings.

Corneal blindness (see Chapters 14 and 19)

Corneal blindness encompasses a wide range of infectious and inflammatory eye diseases; in the developing world, it tends to be related to infectious causes.

The main causes include:

- trachoma
- onchocerciasis
- xerophthalmia (see Chapter 48 for a description of these conditions)
- traumatic corneal abrasion—a major risk factor for microbial keratitis in low- and middle-income countries.

Diabetic retinopathy (DR)

(see Chapters 45 and 46)

Diabetes is a global leading cause of death, disability and economic loss. In South Asia and the Middle East, the prevalence of type 2 diabetes (or diabetes mellitus) is increasing rapidly. This is likely to lead to a high prevalence of DR in this region and subsequent visual impairment unless screening and treatment of retinopathy are undertaken.

Childhood blindness (see Chapter 24)

The number of blind children in the world is approximately 1.4 million. Approximately three-quarters of the world's blind children live in the poorest regions of Africa and Asia. Half a million new cases of childhood corneal blindness are seen each year, and 70% of them are due to vitamin A deficiency, leading to xerophthalmia. Approximately 500 million doses of vitamin A are given annually worldwide, which has greatly reduced childhood mortality and blindness. Paediatric cataract is an important cause of avoidable blindness. Surgical techniques for paediatric cataract have improved, as well as the availability of high-power IOLs that are suitable for children. Retinopathy of prematurity is also emerging as a cause of blindness in urban centres in India, China and other countries in Asia.

KEY POINTS

- Globally, 80% of all visual impairment can be prevented or cured.
- Visual impairment is a major global health issue.
- Globally, uncorrected refractive errors are the main cause of visual impairment; cataracts remain the leading cause of blindness in middle- and low-income countries.

Figure 52.1 Sympathetic innervation causes pupil dilation

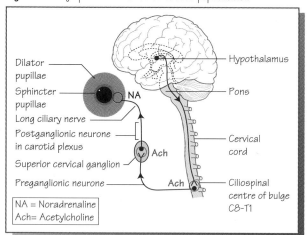

Dilator pupillae
Sphincter pupillae
Long ciliary nerve
Postganglionic neurone in carotid plexus
Superior cervical ganglion
Preganglionic neurone

NA
Ach
Ach

Hypothalamus
Pons
Cervical cord
Ciliospinal centre of bulge C8–T1

NA = Noradrenaline
Ach = Acetylcholine

Figure 52.2 The parasympathetic innervation causes pupil constriction

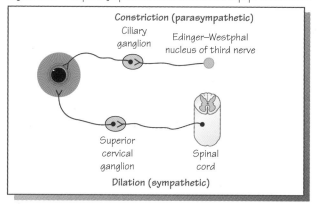

Constriction (parasympathetic)
Ciliary ganglion
Edinger–Westphal nucleus of third nerve
Superior cervical ganglion
Spinal cord
Dilation (sympathetic)

Figure 52.4 Fixed dilated pupil from a posterior communicating aneurysm

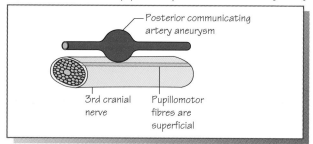

Posterior communicating artery aneurysm
3rd cranial nerve
Pupillomotor fibres are superficial

Figure 52.3 Light reflex pathways

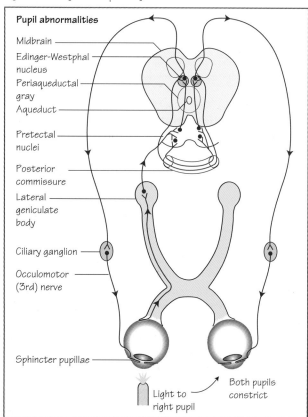

Pupil abnormalities

Midbrain
Edinger-Westphal nucleus
Periaqueductal gray
Aqueduct
Pretectal nuclei
Posterior commissure
Lateral geniculate body
Ciliary ganglion
Occulomotor (3rd) nerve
Sphincter pupillae

Light to right pupil
Both pupils constrict

Figure 52.5 Management of small pupils

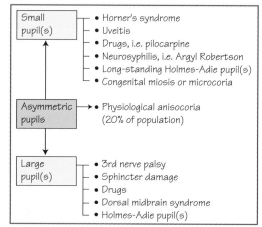

Small pupil(s)
- Horner's syndrome
- Uveitis
- Drugs, i.e. pilocarpine
- Neurosyphilis, i.e. Argyl Robertson
- Long-standing Holmes-Adie pupil(s)
- Congenital miosis or microcoria

Asymmetric pupils
- Physiological anisocoria (20% of population)

Large pupil(s)
- 3rd nerve palsy
- Sphincter damage
- Drugs
- Dorsal midbrain syndrome
- Holmes-Adie pupil(s)

Figure 52.6 Congenital Horner's syndrome

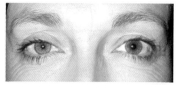

Figure 52.7 Holmes-Adie pupil

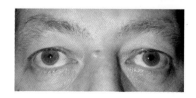

Physiological anisocoria (i.e. unequal pupil size)
This can be distinguished from pathological anisocoria by observing the pupil size in the dark and then in the light – physiological anisocoria, which is usually subtle, should not change dramatically in different levels of illumination (as opposed to Horner's syndrome, which looks worse in the dark). A RAPD indicates serious ophthalmic pathology (most commonly, retinal or optic nerve disease), which warrants immediate referral to an ophthalmologist

Ophthalmology at a Glance, Second Edition. Jane Olver, Lorraine Cassidy, Gurjeet Jutley, and Laura Crawley. © 2014 Jane Olver, Lorraine Cassidy, Gurjeet Jutley and Laura Crawley. Published 2014 by John Wiley & Sons, Ltd. Companion Website: www.ataglanceseries.com/ophthal

You must understand the pupil pathways and the innervation of the pupil.

Aims
- Understand how to assess a patient with abnormal pupils.
- Understand the causes of pupil abnormalities.
- Understand the neuroanatomy of pupillary light reflexes.

Anatomy and physiology
Sympathetic innervation causes pupillary dilation via fibres from the cilio-spinal centre of Bulge via the superior cervical ganglion to the dilator papillae iris muscles (Figure 52.1).

Parasympathetic innervation leads to pupillary constriction via a circular muscle called the *sphincter pupillae*. The pathway of pupillary constriction begins at the Edinger–Westphal nucleus near the oculo-motor nerve nucleus. The fibres enter the orbit with the third cranial nerve (CN III) fibres and synapse at the ciliary ganglion in the poste-rior orbit, then go to the sphincter papillae muscle (Figures 52.2 and 52.3).

Pupil examination
When examining pupils, you need to check for:
- symmetry
- size
- shape
- light response
- near response.

Afferent pupil defect and relative afferent pupillary defect
- An afferent pupil defect (APD) results from damage to the visual pathway anywhere from the retinal ganglion cell layer to the lateral geniculate body, thus causing a reduction in the input (afferent) signal reaching the brainstem when a light is directed at the affected eye. Hence there is a similarly reduced output (efferent) signal reaching the pupil, which consequently constricts to a lesser extent than if it had received a full signal.
- Because of the consensual light reflex, the unaffected pupil will also constrict to an equally lesser extent when the light is directed towards the damaged side.
- Hence, if a light is directed at the better eye, both pupils will constrict fully and equally. If it is then immediately swung over (the 'swinging flash light test') and directed at the affected eye (e.g. an eye with an optic nerve lesion), both pupils will appear to dilate—a relative afferent pupillary defect (RAPD). In fact, what has happened here is that both pupils are constricting but to a lesser degree than when the light was directed at the normal eye, hence they only appear to dilate. When the light is swung back to the better eye, the pupils will constrict.

Fixed dilated pupil
- If a pupil is dilated and doesn't react to light or accommodation, it is important to examine eye movements and levator function in order to exclude a **third nerve palsy**. Note: a unilateral enlarged pupil caused by uncal herniation is a neurosurgical emergency.
- Because of the superficial location of the pupillomotor fibres, a partial third nerve palsy can occur where only the pupil is involved. In such cases, a **tumour** or **posterior communicating artery aneu-rysm** (Figure 52.4) must be excluded.
- A fixed dilated pupil can result from inadvertent or accidental con-tamination of the eye with **cycloplegic agents** such as atropine or cyclopentolate, hence the importance of a detailed history.

- Previous **trauma** or **surgery** where there has been extensive damage to the sphincter pupillae can result in a fixed dilated pupil.
- A fixed semidilated pupil in the presence of a hazy cornea, red eye and pain is seen in **acute angle-closure glaucoma**.

Small pupil (miosis) (Figure 52.5)
- A small pupil in association with a very small amount of ptosis (no more than 2mm—due to paralysis of Müller's muscle) is known as **Horner's syndrome** (Figure 52.6). This results from a lesion of the sympathetic chain anywhere from the hypothalmus to the eye.
- On dimming the lights, the anisocoria will become more obvious as the affected pupil doesn't dilate in the dark as well as its counterpart.
- There may be other associated features such as elevation of the lower lid, which together with the ptosis gives the appearance of enophthalmos, reduced sweating on the ipsilateral side of the face and occasionally conjunctival hyperaemia.
- Horner's syndrome can be confirmed by putting 4% cocaine drops into each eye and observing the pupils 40min later. The normal pupil will dilate, but the Horner's pupil will not.
- Causes of Horner's syndrome include Pancoast's tumour of the lung, thoracic aortic aneurysm, trauma, carotid artery dissection (usually accompanied by neck pain) and central nervous system disease. All patients should be investigated appropriately.
- In **congenital Horner's syndrome**, the iris on the affected side is a different colour—iris heterochromia.
- Contamination of the eye with **pilocarpine** causes miosis.
- Uveitis that has resulted in **posterior synechiae** can result in a small pupil.
- Rarely, **congenital microcoria** can occur.

Light–near dissociation
In some cases, the pupil(s) will accommodate but not react to light. This dissociation of the light and near reflex can occur in various syndromes.
- **Dorsal midbrain** or **Parinaud's syndrome**. This may be due to a lesion (e.g. pinealoma or cranipharyngioma) compressing the pupil-lary light reflex fibres. The pupils may be large and eccentric. Associ-ated features include the absence of an upgaze, upper lid retraction and convergence retraction nystagmus, characterized by rapid conver-gence movements and retraction of both eyes on attempted upgaze.
- **Neurosyphilis** or **Argyll Robertson pupils**. These pupils are small and irregular, do not react to light but react briskly to near stimuli.
- **Holmes–Adie pupil (Figure 52.7)**. This is thought to result from a viral infection; the affected pupil is initially large and eventually may become miosed. There is no reaction to light, and the near reflex is intact but delayed and tonic (the patient should be asked to focus on a near target for at least 1 min before the pupils begin to constrict, and when the patient is then asked to relax his accommodation, the pupils are slow to dilate again). These patients may also have absent tendon reflexes. Both pupils may eventually become involved.
- Patients with **myotonic dystrophy** may have light–near dissociation.
- Patients with **diabetes** may develop a **pupil neuropathy** resulting in light–near dissociation.

KEY POINTS
- A fixed dilated pupil—'surgical third'—must be outruled.
- Unilateral miosis—Horner's syndrome—must be outruled.
- RAPD indicates an optic nerve or retinal disease.

Figure 53.1 Features of optic atrophy and papilloedema. (a) Reduced visual acuity, (b) reduced colour vision or red desaturation, (c) relative afferent pupillary defect and (d) visual field loss

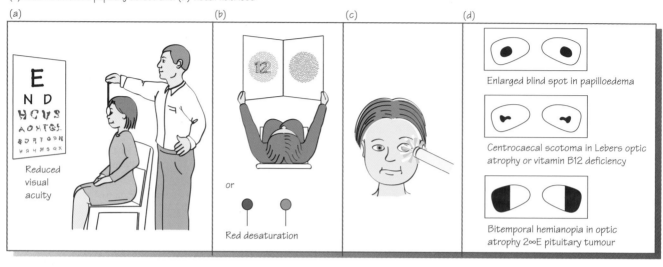

(a) Reduced visual acuity

(b) or Red desaturation

(c)

(d) Enlarged blind spot in papilloedema

Centrocaecal scotoma in Lebers optic atrophy or vitamin B12 deficiency

Bitemporal hemianopia in optic atrophy 2∞E pituitary tumour

Figure 53.2 Multiple sclerosis (MS). (a) (i) Right unilateral optic atrophy in MS, and (ii) normal left disc, (b) (i) acute right papillitis (swollen disc) in MS optic neuritis, and (ii) normal left nerve and (c) (i) a coronal magnetic resonance imaging scan showing demyelination, with a high signal in the right optic nerve, and (ii) a sagittal MRI scan showing demyelination involving the corpus callosum

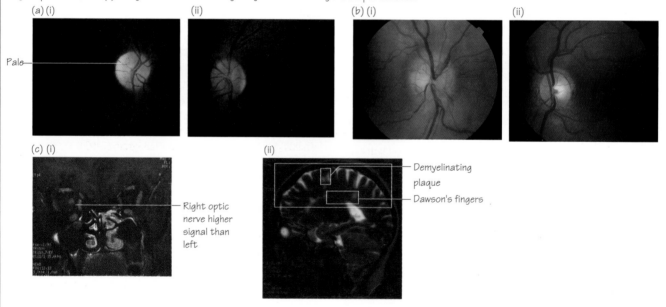

(a) (i) Pale   (ii)   (b) (i)   (ii)

(c) (i) Right optic nerve higher signal than left   (ii) Demyelinating plaque — Dawson's fingers

Figure 53.3 (a and b) Bilateral chronic papilloedema secondary to idiopathic intracranial hypertension (IIH)

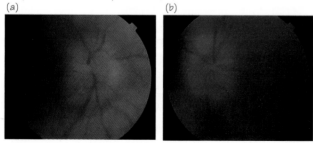

(a)   (b)

Figure 53.4 (a and b) Leber's hereditary optic neuropathy: bilateral involvement. Blurred nasal disc margins and pre-capillary telangiectasis can be seen; typically, discs become swollen in the acute phase

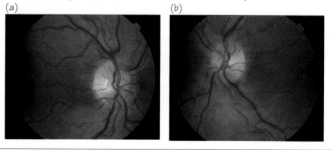

(a)   (b)

Optic nerve disease can be slow and insidious or more acute, and it represents a wide array of pathology, from Leber's hereditary optic neuropathy (LHON) to multiple sclerosis, intracranial tumour and anterior ischaemic optic neuropathy (AION).

Aims
Know the causes of optic atrophy (pale disc) and swollen discs.

Disc swelling
Unilateral disc swelling
Clinical features (Figure 53.1)
- Visual acuity may be normal or reduced.
- Reduced colour vision
- Visual field defect: enlarged blind spot if there is significant swelling, and altitudinal defect if disc swelling is secondary to ischaemic optic neuropathy
- Blurred disc margin ± splinter haemorrhages (Figure 53.2).

Aetiology
- Vascular: for example, AION, central retinal vein or diabetic papillopathy
- Inflammatory: 'papillitis', such as uveitis, sarcoidosis, viral, systemic lupus erythematosus or paranasal sinus disease
- Demyelination: multiple sclerosis—disc swelling may become bilateral (Figure 53.2a and 53.2b). Disc(s) are swollen or normal in the acute phase, and they eventually become pale after recurrent attacks.
- Hereditary: LHON—may become bilateral
- Infiltrative: for example, lymphoma
- Infective: for example, toxoplasmosis, herpes or Lyme disease.

Investigations
- Visual field analysis
- Full blood count (FBC), blood glucose, erythrocyte sedimentation rate (ESR), C-reactive protein, coagulation screen, infective screen (e.g. toxoplasmosis and *Borelia* titres), autoantibody screen
- Blood is sent for analysis for Leber's mutation if suspected.
- Neuroimaging if demyelination or a compressive lesion is suspected. Magnetic resonance imaging (MRI) of the brain and optic nerves should be requested (Figure 53.2c).
- Lumbar puncture if demyelination, neurosarcoidosis or lymphoma is suspected.

Bilateral disc swelling and papilloedema
Clinical features
- Visual acuity may be normal or severely reduced.
- Patients with papilloedema may complain of episodes of unilateral or bilateral transient visual loss lasting for a few seconds. These are transient visual obscurations (TVOs) and can be precipitated by changes in posture.
- Colour vision is often reduced.
- Enlarged blind spot if the swelling is significant; it will be normal in mild cases.

Aetiology
- Raised intracranial pressure: space-occupying lesion, hydrocephalus, idiopathic intracranial hypertension (IIH)
- Malignant hypertension
- Diabetic papillopathy
- Infiltrative papilloedema (Figure 53.3), such as lymphoma
- Toxic, such as ethambutol.

Investigations
- Blood pressure; Glucose, FBC and differential white cell count, U&E, creatinine and ESR; Neuroimaging; Lumbar puncture if the MRI is normal and IIH is suspected; Visual fields (to monitor blind spot).

Table 53.1 Leber's hereditary optic neuropathy

- A hereditary optic neuropathy affecting young males 20–30 years old
- Mitochondrial inheritance (i.e. passed via mitochondrial DNA) passed through the female side of the family in most cases
- Often smokers
- Presents with:
  - Subacute painless loss of central vision in one or both eyes
  - Second eye involved within weeks to months
  - Centrocaecal scotoma
  - Typical circumpapillary telangiectatic microangiopathy
- The primary mutation has prognostic implications:
  - 11778: 2–17% recovery
  - 3460: 15–30% recovery
  - 14484: 37–50% recovery
- Treatment : none, advise to stop smoking.

Optic atrophy and neuropathy
Clinical features
- VA is reduced but can be normal, depending on the degree of optic atrophy.
- Relative afferent pupillary defect.
- Disc pallor. In severe optic atrophy, the entire disc may be pale; in many cases, only part of the disc (e.g. the temporal part) will be affected, and subtle disc pallor will be missed if both discs are not compared.

Aetiology
- **Hereditary:**
  - Autosomal dominant optic atrophy: Affected family members may vary considerably in abnormalities.
  - Autosomal recessive optic atrophy: poor visual acuity
  - LHON (Figure 53.4 and Table 53.1).
- **Retinal dystrophy:**
  - Cone dystrophy: very poor acuity, markedly reduced colour vision, photophobia, central scotoma, nystagmus and typical ERG
  - Retinitis pigmentosa: typical retinal appearance, constricted visual fields and characteristic electroretinogram (ERG)
- **Vascular:** central retinal artery occlusion see chapter 48.
- **Nutritional or toxic:** vitamin B_{12} deficiency (gradual bilateral visual loss associated with pins and needles in hands and feet, poor diet, reduced colour vision and centrocaecal scotoma), tobacco–alcohol amblyopia or drugs (e.g. ethambutol or chloramphenicol).
- **Inflammatory:** sarcoidosis, polyarteritis nodosa, contiguous sinus disease—more commonly present with disc swelling.
- **Demyelination:** may have past history of typical attacks of optic neuritis, and may have other neurological symptoms. It is a common cause.
- **Compressive:** optic nerve glioma or meningioma, orbital tumour or intracranial tumour.

Investigations
- Formal visual field testing
- Visual evoked response or potential (VER or VEP)
- ERG
- Relevant blood tests depending on clinical history (e.g. vitamin B_{12} and folate levels in a patient who is a vegan and has bilateral optic atrophy with glove and stocking paraesthesia)
- Neuroimaging: MRI optic nerves and brain.

KEY POINTS
- Rule out malignant hypertension in papilloedema.
- *Urgent* CT brain if headache, nausea, papilloedema and normal BP.
- MRI if demyelination is suspected.

Figure 54.1 Neuroanatomy of the 3rd, 4th, 6th and 7th cranial nerves

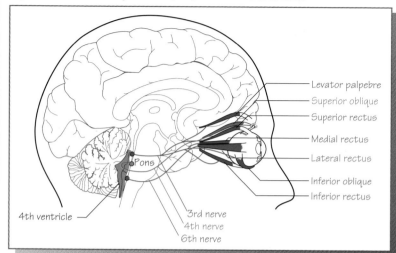

Levator palpebre
Superior oblique
Superior rectus
Medial rectus
Lateral rectus
Inferior oblique
Inferior rectus

Pons
4th ventricle
3rd nerve
4th nerve
6th nerve

Figure 54.2 Right 3rd cranial nerve palsy

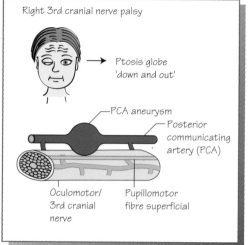

Right 3rd cranial nerve palsy

Ptosis globe 'down and out'

PCA aneurysm
Posterior communicating artery (PCA)

Oculomotor/ 3rd cranial nerve
Pupillomotor fibre superficial

Figure 54.3 Right 4th cranial nerve palsy

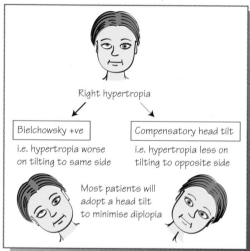

Right hypertropia

Bielchowsky +ve	Compensatory head tilt
i.e. hypertropia worse on tilting to same side	i.e. hypertropia less on tilting to opposite side

Most patients will adopt a head tilt to minimise diplopia

Figure 54.4 Right 6th cranial nerve palsy

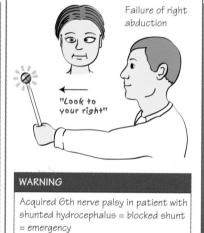

Failure of right abduction

"Look to your right"

WARNING

Acquired 6th nerve palsy in patient with shunted hydrocephalus = blocked shunt = emergency

Figure 54.5 Right 7th cranial nerve palsy

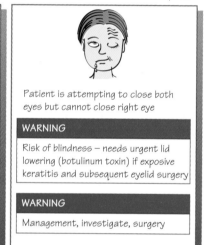

Patient is attempting to close both eyes but cannot close right eye

WARNING

Risk of blindness – needs urgent lid lowering (botulinum toxin) if exposive keratitis and subsequent eyelid surgery

WARNING

Management, investigate, surgery

Figure 54.6 Right internuclear ophthalmoplegia (INO)

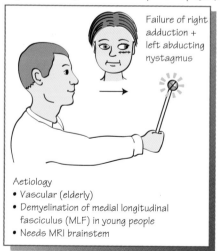

Failure of right adduction + left abducting nystagmus

Aetiology
• Vascular (elderly)
• Demyelination of medial longitudinal fasciculus (MLF) in young people
• Needs MRI brainstem

Figure 54.7 Nystagmus (e.g. albinism)

Albino - this child's parents are coloured. Notice the pale skin and white eye lashes

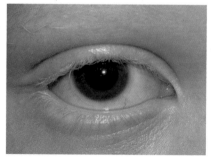

Albinism
Signs: • infantile nystagmus
• decreased VA and photophobia
• iris transillumination
2 types   i) oculocutaneous: hair, skin, eyes
Tyrosinase +ve – some pigment as adult
Tyrosinase –ve – never pigment, typical 'albino'
ii) ocular: eye pigment affected, hair, skin are normal
Needs visual aids, tinted spectacles for glare, sun/skin advice, genetic counselling

Ophthalmology at a Glance, Second Edition. Jane Olver, Lorraine Cassidy, Gurjeet Jutley, and Laura Crawley. © 2014 Jane Olver, Lorraine Cassidy, Gurjeet Jutley and Laura Crawley. Published 2014 by John Wiley & Sons, Ltd. Companion Website: www.ataglanceseries.com/ophthal

Aim

Describe clinical features of third, fourth, fifth and seventh cranial nerve palsies, internuclear ophthalmoplegia (INO), gaze palsies and nystagmus. The neuroanatomy of these cranial nerves is shown in Figure 54.1.

Third nerve palsy (Figure 54.2)

Symptoms

- Double vision—horizontal and/or vertical
- Droopy lid
- Enlarged pupil
- Headache. Note painful third nerve with pupil involvement—exclude a posterior communicating artery aneurysm as soon as possible.

Signs

- Ptosis
- Exotropia and hypotropia (globe appears down and out)
- Fixed dilated pupil
- Limitation of elevation, depression and adduction

May present with any of these or a combination.

Aetiology

- Ischaemic or vascular (usually pupil sparing due to the anatomy of the pupillomotor fibres, and referred to as a 'medical third'): diabetes mellitus (DM), hypertension, vasculitis or migraine
- Compressive lesion (pupil nearly always involved, and referred to as a 'surgical third'): posterior communicating artery aneurysm or tumour
- Trauma
- Congenital third.

Fourth nerve palsy (Figure 54.3)

Symptoms

Double vision—vertical.

Signs

- Head tilt opposite to the side of the lesion.
- Hypertropia on the affected side.
- Limitation of eye movement down and to the right if left fourth nerve palsy, and vice versa.
- Positive Bielchowsky's sign, that is, the hypertropia on the affected side gets worse on tilting the head to the same side.

Aetiology

- Trauma is the most common cause of fourth nerve palsy as this nerve has the longest intracranial course, is very slender and runs under the tentorial edge. Trauma may result in bilateral fourths.
- Ischaemic or vascular: DM, hypertension or vasculitis
- Compressive lesion (e.g. intracranial tumour)
- Congenital.

Fifth nerve palsy

Corneal anaesthesia.

Sixth nerve palsy (Figure 54.4)

Symptoms

Double vision—horizontal especially at distance.

Signs

- Esotropia; it is worse for distance.
- Limitation of abduction of the affected eye.

Aetiology

- Vascular or ischaemic: DM, hypertension, or vasculitis
- Invading intracranial or nasopharyngeal tumour
- Trauma (e.g. fractured skull base).

Seventh nerve palsy (Figure 54.5)

Symptoms

- Inability to close eyelid (lagophthalmos) and facial weakness
- Watery eye (due to weakness of orbicularis oculi)
- Sore red eye (due to corneal exposure)
- Blurred vision secondary to exposure keratitis
- Drooling.

Signs

- Ipsilateral facial muscle weakness, involving the frontalis in lower motor neurone lesions. The frontalis is spared in upper motor neurone lesions.
- Lower lid ectropion secondary to orbicularis oculi weakness.
- Corneal exposure may vary from superficial punctate erosions to corneal abrasion, and it must be treated urgently to prevent abscess formation and endophthalmitis.

Aetiology

- Viral or idiopahtic, such as Bell's palsy (usually improves spontaneously) or Ramsay–Hunt syndrome (herpes simplex infection)
- Compressive lesion: intracranial tumour, such as acoustic neuroma (may have associated fifth, sixth and eighth nerve palsy) or parotid tumour
- Vascular or ischaemic: DM, hypertension or vasculitis
- Inflammation (e.g. sarcoidosis).

Internuclear ophthalmoplegia (Figure 54.6)

Symptoms

- Horizontal diplopia
- Inability to coordinate eye movements.

Signs

- Failure to adduct the ipsilateral eye
- Abducting nystagmus of the contralateral eye.

Nystagmus (Figure 54.7)

This is involuntary rhythmic to-and-fro oscillation of the eyes.

Symptoms

- Congenital nystagmus is asymptomatic.
- Acquired nystagmus may cause oscillopsia, a sensation of rapid movement or oscillation of the visual environment. Patients describe it as though looking at an old black-and-white film where everything flickers or wobbles; others notice only blurred vision, especially with gaze-evoked nystagmus.

> **WARNING**
>
> ▶ Refer any patient with nystagmus for prompt assessment by a neuro-ophthalmologist to exclude intracranial SOL.

> **KEY POINTS**
>
> - Painful third—posterior communicating artery aneurysm.
> - Traumatic sixth—basal skull fracture.
> - Internuclear ophthalmoplegia—demyelination.

Figure 55.1 Neuroanatomy of the visual pathway

Left temporal field
Left nasal field
Right nasal field
Right temporal field

Nasal retina
Temporal retina
Optic nerve
Von Willbrand's knee
Optic tract
Chiasm

Lateral geniculate body
Meyer's loop
Inferior horn of lateral ventricle
Optic radiation

Occipital visual cortex

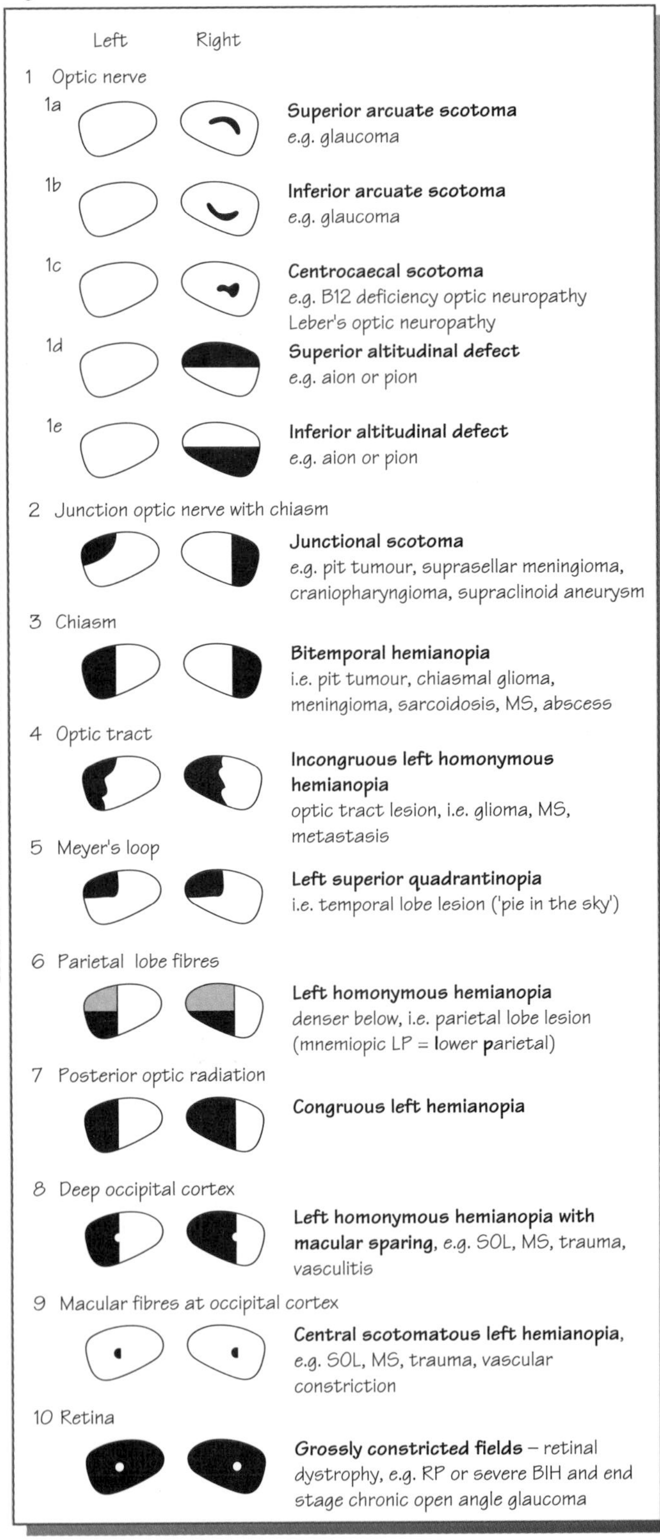

Tumours

Figure 55.3 Types of tumour that affect the visual pathway

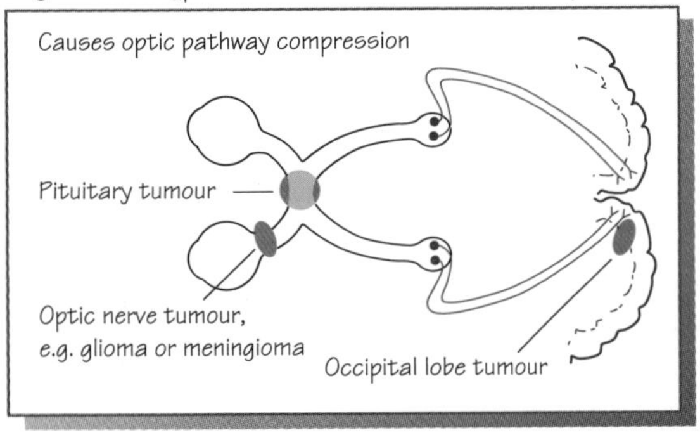

Causes optic pathway compression

Pituitary tumour

Optic nerve tumour, e.g. glioma or meningioma

Occipital lobe tumour

A detailed knowledge of the neuroanatomy of the visual pathway can help the clinician to localize lesions from the field defect found

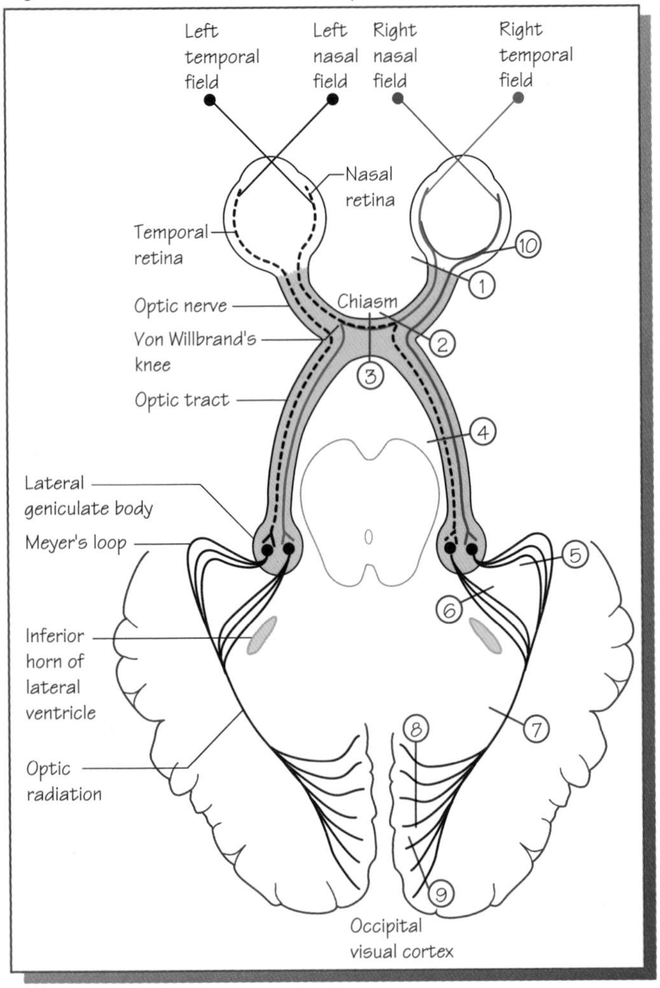

Figure 55.2 Associated visual field defects

Left   Right

1 Optic nerve

1a **Superior arcuate scotoma** e.g. glaucoma

1b **Inferior arcuate scotoma** e.g. glaucoma

1c **Centrocaecal scotoma** e.g. B12 deficiency optic neuropathy Leber's optic neuropathy

1d **Superior altitudinal defect** e.g. aion or pion

1e **Inferior altitudinal defect** e.g. aion or pion

2 Junction optic nerve with chiasm

Junctional scotoma e.g. pit tumour, suprasellar meningioma, craniopharyngioma, supraclinoid aneurysm

3 Chiasm

Bitemporal hemianopia i.e. pit tumour, chiasmal glioma, meningioma, sarcoidosis, MS, abscess

4 Optic tract

Incongruous left homonymous hemianopia optic tract lesion, i.e. glioma, MS, metastasis

5 Meyer's loop

Left superior quadrantinopia i.e. temporal lobe lesion ('pie in the sky')

6 Parietal lobe fibres

Left homonymous hemianopia denser below, i.e. parietal lobe lesion (mnemiopic LP = lower parietal)

7 Posterior optic radiation

Congruous left hemianopia

8 Deep occipital cortex

Left homonymous hemianopia with macular sparing, e.g. SOL, MS, trauma, vasculitis

9 Macular fibres at occipital cortex

Central scotomatous left hemianopia, e.g. SOL, MS, trauma, vascular constriction

10 Retina

Grossly constricted fields – retinal dystrophy, e.g. RP or severe BIH and end stage chronic open angle glaucoma

Ophthalmology at a Glance, Second Edition. Jane Olver, Lorraine Cassidy, Gurjeet Jutley, and Laura Crawley. © 2014 Jane Olver, Lorraine Cassidy, Gurjeet Jutley and Laura Crawley. Published 2014 by John Wiley & Sons, Ltd. Companion Website: www.ataglanceseries.com/ophthal

Please also refer to Chapter 6, 'Examination of Visual Fields'. You should know the type of visual field to perform to optimally detect the type of visual field defect.

Aims

- Understand the neuroanatomy of the various visual field defects (Figures 55.1 and 55.2).
- Recognize the causes of different field defects.

Visual field defects

The most common visual field defects encountered in clinical practice include homonymous hemianopia, altitudinal field defect, bitemporal hemianopia, grossly constricted fields and enlarged blind spots.

Note obvious clues that will help you (e.g. a hemiparesis)—this patient is most likely to have an ipsilateral hemianopia as the result of a lesion in the contralateral cortex.

Optic nerve

A unilateral optic nerve lesion can result in various unilateral field defects depending on the nature of the lesion. The shape of field defect can give a clue to the diagnosis. For example:
- Glaucomatous cupping can result in an **arcuate scotoma** of the superior (Figure 55.2, 1a) or inferior field (Figure 55.2, 1b).
- Vitamin B$_{12}$ deficiency can result in a **centrocaecal scotoma** (Figure 55.2, 1c).
- Anterior ischaemic optic neuropathy (a swollen disc can be seen in the acute phase) and posterior ischaemic optic neuropathy (the disc will look normal in the acute phase) can result in an **altitudinal field defect**. This can be superior (Figure 55.2, 1d) or inferior (Figure 55.2, 1e), depending on which vessels are involved.
- Complete severing of the optic nerve (e.g. as a result of trauma) will cause **complete ipsilateral visual field loss**.

Junction optic nerve with chiasm

Because of the arrangement of nerve fibres in the optic nerve and chiasm, a lesion pressing on the visual pathway at the junction of the intracranial optic nerve and the chiasm can produce a characteristic field defect (Figure 55.2, 2), known as a **junctional scotoma**. Such a field defect results because the lesion compresses both fibres from the nasal fibres (serving the temporal visual field) of the ipsilateral optic nerve and the inferonasal fibres (superotemporal field) from the contralateral eye in Willebrand's knee.

Chiasm

A lesion pressing on the optic chiasm, such as a pituitary tumour (Figure 55.3), will result in damage to the nasal fibres from both eyes as they cross the midline, and therefore results in a **bitemporal hemianopia** (Figure 55.2, 3). Early on, if the lesion is only minimally compressing the chiasm, the field defect will be very subtle and may be picked up only by using a red target (the individual will have red desaturation in the affected field—this is true for all subtle lesions).

Optic tract

A lesion of the optic tract involves the temporal fibres (nasal field) from the ipsilateral eye and the crossed nasal fibres (temporal field) from the contralateral eye. A lesion completely destroying, for example, the right optic tract will result in a complete left **homonymous hemianopia**. However, most optic tract lesions are partial, and because corresponding fibres from the nasal and retinal fields are not so close together in the tract, the homonymous hemianopia produced is incongruous (i.e. the hemi-field defect from the right eye is not an identical shape to that of the left) (Figure 55.2, 4).

Meyer's loop

A lesion of the optic radiation in the temporal lobe will affect Meyer's loop, which contains fibres representing the inferior quadrant of the ipsilateral temporal retina, and the contralateral nasal retina. This results in a **superior homonymous quadrantanopia**, sometimes referred to as a 'pie in the sky' defect (Figure 55.2, 5).

Parietal lobe

A lesion in the parietal lobe may affect the fibres from the superior quadrants of the ipsilateral temporal and contralateral nasal retina, giving rise to an **inferior homonymous quadrantanopia** or a homonymous hemianopia that is denser below than above (Figure 55.2, 6).

Optic radiation to occipital cortex

Any unilateral lesion affecting the more anterior portion of the occipital cortex will give rise to a homonymous hemianopia. Because of the close proximity of the cells representing the corresponding retinal points, the hemianopia will be **congruous** (Figure 55.2, 7), unlike the incongruous hemianopia seen with an optic tract lesion (the more posterior the lesion, the more congruous the field defect). Because the macula has a large representation in the occipital cortex, and a dual blood supply, the central 5° of vision is maintained in an anterior cortical lesion—**macular sparing** (Figure 55.2, 8).

Macular fibres at occipital cortex

A posterior lesion affecting one side of the occipital cortex will result in a **homonymous hemianopic scotomatous** field defect (Figure 55.2, 9).

Retina

Retinal disease can grossly restrict the visual fields, as can advanced chronic open-angle glaucoma (Figure 55.2, 10).

KEY POINTS

- Bitemporal hemianopia indicates a chiasmal lesion—most commonly a pituitary tumour.
- Left homonymous hemianopia indicates a right cortical brain lesion.
- Altitudinal field defect is typical of anterior ischaemic optic neuropathy.

Figure 56.1 Giant cell arteritis (GCA). A sclerotic, non-pulsatile superficial temporal artery (STA) (a) is an indicator that the patient may have GCA if he presents with visual symptoms. The visual symptoms are not attributed to involvement of the STA; rather, this is a marker of disease and increases the likelihood that the ophthalmic vessel is affected (b)

(a)

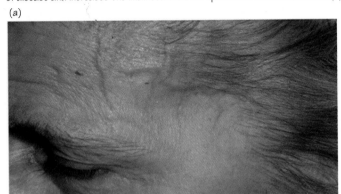

(b)

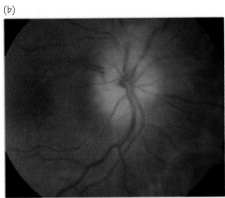

Table 56.1 Immune-related systemic vasculitides and the eye. Since the eye is a vascular organ, it can be affected by a group of disorders with the hallmark of inflammatory destruction of either arteries or veins (or, indeed, both). Symptoms are attributed to the specific vascular involvement, and characterization is based on vessel size

Type of vasculitis	Clinical features	Relevant investigations
Large vessel disease		
Behçet's disease	Recurrent oral ulcerations, skin lesions (including erythema nodusum), genital ulceration, uveitis, arthritis, intestinal involvement and vascular occlusion	Clinical diagnosis
Takayasu's	Granulomatous inflammation of different parts of the aorta leads to various clinical manifestations (e.g. hypertension secondary to renal artery stenosis)	Magnetic resonance angiogram
Medium-vessel disease		
Polyarteritis nodosa (i.e. Kussmaul disease)	Association with hepatitis B infection; symptoms relate to organs affected by the vessel involvement (i.e. cutaneous venous involvement leads to livedo reticularis)	p-ANCA, tissue biopsy
Kawasaki disease	Fever, erythema of lips and oral cavity, truncal rash, swelling of hands and feet, conjunctival injection and cervical lymphadenopathy	Clinical diagnosis
Thromboangiitis obliterans (i.e. Berger's disease)	Progressive inflammation and thrombosis of vessels and feet; strong association with smoking	Angiograms
Small-vessel disease		
Allergic granulomatosis (i.e. Churg–Strauss syndrome)	Pulmonary involvement (asthma, pulmonary infiltrates and para-nasal infiltrates) and mono- and polyneuropathy	p-ANCA, eosinophilia
Wegener's granulomatosis	Systems involved include renal (progressive glomurelo-nephritis), pulmonary (tracheal stenosis, pulmonary nodules and infiltrates), upper airways (saddle nose defects, epitaxis), cutaneous (purpura), arthritic (swelling), nervous (sensory neuropathy) and ocular (scleritis)	c-ANCA, biopsy

Giant cell arteritis (GCA) is an ophthalmic and medical emergency.

Aims

- Appreciate that ocular diagnosis of GCA can be lifesaving.
- Be aware of GCA as a diagnosis, and investigate it appropriately.

GCA

- GCA is a very important type of vasculitis manifesting in the eye. It is a disease that enables the student to appreciate how an ophthalmic diagnosis can be lifesaving. GCA is very commonly seen in eye casualty, and all physicians need to be able to manage it.
- GCA predominantly affects medium and large-sized arteries, particularly the main branches of the aorta, the primary and secondary branches, and the superficial temporal, ophthalmic, posterior ciliary and vertebral arteries (Figure 56.1a).
- GCA is between two and six times more common in women and is almost always seen in patients older than 50 (incidence is 15–25 per 100 000 per year in those over 50 years).

Pathology

- GCA is characterized by granulomatous inflammation at the level of the internal elastic lamina, with an influx of macrophages, lymphocytes, fibroblasts and occasionally multinucleated giant cells (Figure 56.1b).
- These manifest as 'skip lesions', and areas adjacent to these remain unaffected.
- The inflammatory infiltrate and subsequent intimal hyperplasia can limit perfusion to the distal tissue, and ischaemia ensues.

Ophthalmic manifestations

- Unilateral visual disturbance (transient or permanent) is due to central retinal artery occlusion or arteritic anterior ischaemic neuropathy (AAION).
- Double vision is due to cranial nerve palsies.

Systemic associations

Polymyalgia rheumatica (PR) represents a systemic manifestation of the same underlying pathological process, causing distress by pain and morning stiffness in the neck, shoulder and pelvis. Ischaemic changes are not as readily seen as with GCA, and PR responds to low-dose steroids.

Clinical features

Symptoms

- Neuro-ophthalmic:
  - headache and scalp tenderness (compromised superficial temporal artery)
  - hair loss and scalp ischaemia
  - diplopia
  - jaw claudication (ischaemia to the masseter)
- Systemic:
  - myalgia
  - anorexia
  - weight loss

Signs

- Point tenderness over the temporal artery.
- White and swollen optic nerve head, cotton wool spots, haemorrhages, relative afferent pupil defect and visual field defects (AAION or vein occlusions).
- Asymmetrical pulses and blood pressure readings (involvement of the subclavian artery).
- Extreme cases will cause aortic dissection, transient ischemic attack or strokes.

Investigations and diagnosis (Table 56.1)

- Acute phase response proteins (but may be normal)
  - a large American study has shown that in the absence of another cause, raised levels of both C-reactive protein (CRP) **and** the erythrocyte sedimentation rate (ESR) are strong predictors of disease.
- Thrombocytosis.
- Liver function test.
- Temporal artery biopsy (TAB) shows necrotizing vasculitis, but may be negative due to the nature of skip lesions.
- Ultrasound shows up arterial wall oedema as hypo-echoic 'halos'; but this investigation is more a research tool, rather than being used readily clinically.
- Overall: if clinically suspicious and all results are negative, treat the patient for active disease.

Treatment

- Usually visual loss cannot be halted in the involved eye, and treatment is geared to prevent contralaterally morbidity and indeed mortality. Oral glucocorticoids are the mainstay of treatment (initially prednisolone 1 mg/kg), and most patients are treated and weaned off over a year.
- Unfortunately, there are multiple side effects associated with steroid use, including fluid retention, hypertension, hyperglycaemia, immune suppression, osteoporosis and psychoses. Hence, treating any inflammatory condition in the long run should involve steroid-sparing agents.
- The evidence for steroid-sparing agents is fairly inconclusive. The most investigated agent is methotrexate, and one meta-analysis revealed that administrating a low dose late on in the disease reduces relapses. Poor results have been seen with all other agents, particularly infliximab.
- Aspirin reduces the risk of CVA.

KEY POINTS

- ESR upper limits of normal: men = age / 2; women = (age + 10) / 2.
- Do **not** hold off steroids whilst awaiting the biopsy result.
- Jaw claudication is very characteristic of GCA.
- Always consider GCA as a diagnosis in patients over 50, but do not order ESR or CRP without clinical suspicion, as a patient may receive high-dose steroids incorrectly based on an intermediate result.

Appendix 1: Red eye—signs and symptoms of different causes

Signs and symptoms	Conjunctivitis	Subconjunctival haemorrhage	Corneal abrasion	Allergy	Iritis	Acute glaucoma	Corneal ulcer
History	Family or friend	Trauma, hypertension incidental	Injury	Hay fever, asthma, eczema	Nil or other inflammatory disease	Change of lighting worse in dim light	Contact lens, injury
Sensation	Grittiness	None, mild irritation	Pain, photophobia	Itching	Pain, photophobia	Pain, photophobia, nausea	Pain, photophobia
Vision	Normal	Normal	Decreased (if central)	Normal	Decreased	Decreased	Decreased
Discharge	Purulent or clear	None	Tearing	Mucus	Tearing	Tearing	Tearing and mucopurulent
Pupillary light reflex	Brisk	Brisk	Brisk	Brisk	Normal	Mid-dilated and fixed	May be sluggish
Conjunctival injection	Diffuse, tarsal area	Localized, bright red	Diffuse	Diffuse, tarsal area	Circumcorneal	Diffuse	Circumcorneal
Corneal appearance	Clear	Clear	Stains with fluorescein	Clear	Keratic precipitates	Cloudy cornea	Stains with fluorescein
Intraocular pressure	Normal	Normal	Normal	Normal	Normal or elevated	Markedly elevated	Normal or elevated
Basic management	Hygiene, may rarely require topical antibiotics	Reassurance, check blood pressure	Topical antibiotics	Topical antihistamine	Ophthalmic referral	Urgent Ophthalmic referral	Ophthalmic referral

Ophthalmology at a Glance, Second Edition. Jane Olver, Lorraine Cassidy, Gurjeet Jutley, and Laura Crawley. © 2014 Jane Olver, Lorraine Cassidy, Gurjeet Jutley and Laura Crawley. Published 2014 by John Wiley & Sons, Ltd. Companion Website: www.ataglanceseries.com/ophthal

Appendix 2: The layers of the retina

Number	Layer	Description
i	Choriocapillaris	Fenestrated vessels that give an early choroidal flush seen on fundus fluorescein angiography
ii	Bruch's membrane	Made up of five layers, including the basement membrane of the RPE and endothelium of the capillaries of the capillary layer
iii	Retinal pigment epithelium (RPE)	Role includes absorption of light, storing and releasing vitamin A and aiding turnover of outer segments of photoreceptors
iv	Photoreceptors	Two types of cells make up the photoreceptor layer. The rods process vision in dim light and in the periphery. Cones can resolve fine details and colours.
v	Outer limiting membrane	Outer process of the Müller cell, which is a supporting cell group of the retina
vi	Outer nuclear layer	Nuclei of rod and cone cells
vii	Outer plexiform layer	Synapse between rod and cones with bipolar cells
viii	Inner nuclear layer	Nuclei of bipolar cells; this cell group is an intermediary cell group that synapses with photoreceptor and ganglion cells.
ix	Inner plexiform layer	Synapse between bipolar cells and ganglion cells
x	Ganglion cell layer	Nuclei of ganglion cells. These axons make a 90° turn when they reach the inner surface of the retina.
xi	Nerve fibre layer	Axons of ganglion cells
xii	Inner limiting membrane	Termination of the Müller cells

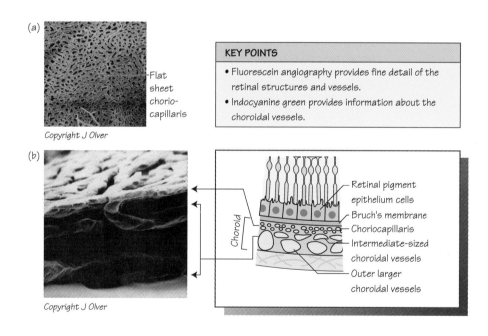

(a)

Flat sheet chorio-capillaris

Copyright J Olver

KEY POINTS

- Fluorescein angiography provides fine detail of the retinal structures and vessels.
- Indocyanine green provides information about the choroidal vessels.

(b)

Copyright J Olver

Retinal pigment epithelium cells
Bruch's membrane
Choriocapillaris
Intermediate-sized choroidal vessels
Outer larger choroidal vessels

Choroid

Ophthalmology at a Glance, Second Edition. Jane Olver, Lorraine Cassidy, Gurjeet Jutley, and Laura Crawley. © 2014 Jane Olver, Lorraine Cassidy, Gurjeet Jutley and Laura Crawley. Published 2014 by John Wiley & Sons, Ltd. Companion Website: www.ataglanceseries.com/ophthal

Appendix 3: Pharmacological intraocular pressure (IOP)-lowering agents—mechanism of action and side effects

Agent	Dose	Action	Side effects
Prostaglandin analogues and prostamide			
Bimatoprost (Lumigan®)	Once daily	Potentiates uveoscleral pathway and conventional pathway	Periocular skin pigmentation
Latanoprost (Xalatan®)	Preferably nocte		Eyelash growth
Tafluprost (Saflutan®)	Unoprostone twice daily		Iris pigmentation
Travoprost (Travatan®)			Few systemic side effects
Unoprostone (Rescula®)			
Beta (β) blockers			
Beta 1 selective	Twice daily	Decreases aqueous production	Bronchospasm
Betaxolol (Betoptic)			Bradycardia
Non-selective	Once daily in gel form		Hypotension, especially nocturnal
Levobunolol (Betagan)			
Timolol			
Alpha (α) agonists			
Alpha-2 selective			
Apraclonidine (Iopidine®)	Apraclonidine 2–3 times daily	Decreases aqueous production	Contact dermatitis
Brimonidine (Alphagan®)	Brimonidine twice daily	Brimonidine also increases uveoscleral ouflow.	Follicular conjunctivitis
			Monoamine oxidase inhibitor reaction
Carbonic anhydrase inhibitors			
Topical	3× daily as monotherapy	Decreases aqueous production	Sulphonamide allergy: anaphylaxis
Brinzolamide 1% (Azopt®)			Steven–Johnson syndrome
Dorzolamide 2% (Trusopt®)	2× daily in combination		Bone marrow depression
Systemic	Acetazolamide		Metallic taste
Acetazolamide (Diamox®)	250 mg 4× daily		Metabolic acidosis
	250 mg slow-release capsule twice daily.		Hypokalaemia paraesthesia
	Intra-venous route		Tinnitus
	500 mg stat		Renal calculi, depression
Parasympathomimetics			
Direct acting	4× daily	Increases aqueous outflow	Meiosis
Pilocarpine		Direct action on longitudinal ciliary muscle	Accommodative spasm Pseudomyopia
			Brow ache
Combination therapy		Combines the effect of the two agents	
Lumigan and timolol (Ganforte®)			
Travatan and timolol (Duotrav®)			
Xalatan and timolol (Xalacom®)			
Azopt and timolol (Azarga®)		Aim is improved compliance.	
Trusopt and timolol (Cosopt®)			

Ophthalmology at a Glance, Second Edition. Jane Olver, Lorraine Cassidy, Gurjeet Jutley, and Laura Crawley. © 2014 Jane Olver, Lorraine Cassidy, Gurjeet Jutley and Laura Crawley. Published 2014 by John Wiley & Sons, Ltd. Companion Website: www.ataglanceseries.com/ophthal

Appendix 4: Optical coherence tomography (OCT) reports

Appendix 4.1   Normal disc

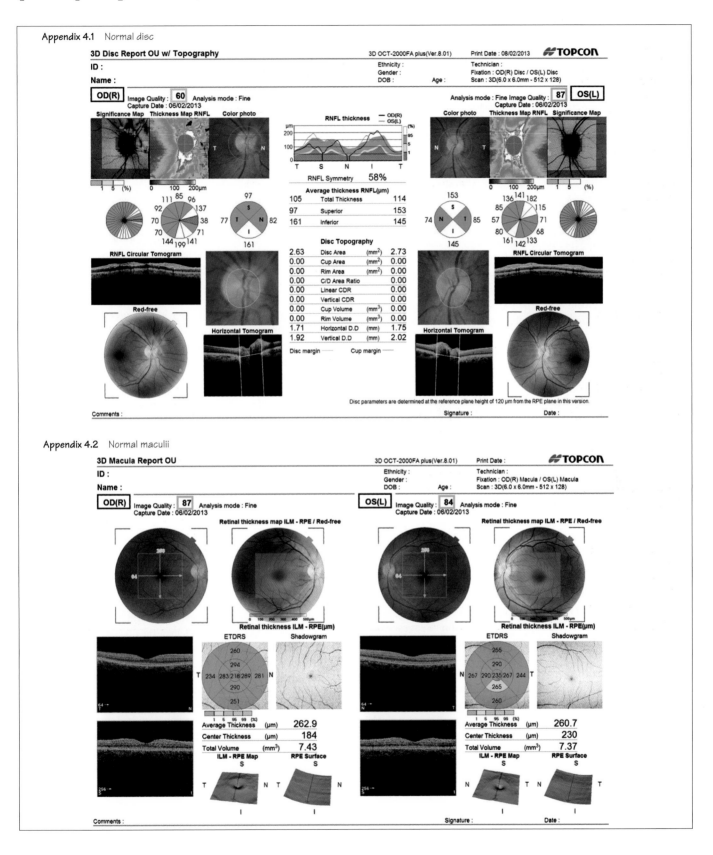

Appendix 4.2   Normal maculii

Ophthalmology at a Glance, Second Edition. Jane Olver, Lorraine Cassidy, Gurjeet Jutley, and Laura Crawley. © 2014 Jane Olver, Lorraine Cassidy, Gurjeet Jutley and Laura Crawley. Published 2014 by John Wiley & Sons, Ltd. Companion Website: www.ataglanceseries.com/ophthal

Appendix 5: Important clinical trials in AMD

The **Macular Photocoagulation Study (MPS)** was the first important study in the treatment of AMD. The study looked at three distinct locations of classic neovascular membranes:
- Extra-foveal lesions were treated with argon photocoagulation; patients were recruited from 1979 to 1984.
- Juxta-foveal lesions were treated with krypton laser photocoagulation; recruitment was from 1981 to 1987.
- Patients with subfoveal lesions were recruited from 1986 to 1990.

The study group concluded that patients in the first two groups benefited from laser, if strict criteria were adhered to.

Treatment of AMD with Photodynamic Therapy (TAP): one-year results were published in 1999. The principle of PDT is harnessing the energy transfer produced from the interaction of light (red light of wavelength 693 nm), oxygen and intravenously administered photosensitizer (usually verteporfin) to enable a local destructive effect. The vascular membranes take up the photosensitizer, thus enabling selective treatment. The energy transfer creates an oxygen-free radical molecule, which results in local damage to the endothelium of the choroidal neovascular membrane. The TAP study showed that patients with predominantly classic sub-foveal lesions had the greatest treatment benefit when treated with PDT.

Verteporfin in Photodynamic Therapy (VIP) was a double-masked, placebo-controlled, randomized multicentre trial that investigated PDT treatment of occult CNVM. Results were published between 2001 and 2003. At 12 months, there was no difference in both groups; hence, PDT has no role in managing large occult CNVM. Currently PDT has a limited role, being used in the management of chronic CSR, choroidal haemangioma, and in combination with intravitreal anti-VEGF agents for IPCV.

MARINA (Minimally Classic/Occult Trial 2006 of the Anti-VEGF Antibody Ranibizumab in the Treatment of Neovascular Age-Related Macular Degeneration) compared monthly ranibizumab with placebo in participants with occult membranes. 34% of those treated with 0.5 mg gained 15 letters, compared to 5% in controls.

ANCHOR (Anti-VEGF Antibody Trial 2006 for the Treatment of Predominantly classic Choroidal Neovascularization in Age-Related Macular Degeneration) compared monthly ranibizumab with PDT in classic neovascularization. 40% receiving 0.5 mg gained 15 letters, compared with 6% in the PDT group.

The **Prospective OCT Study with Lucentis for Neovascular AMD (PrONTO) 2009 trial** aimed to guide when to re-treat. The 2-year results were published after ANCHOR and MARINA in 2006. In the first year, patients were assessed and treated on a monthly basis. For the following year, patients were re-treated only if there was an increase in central retinal thickness, as shown on OCT. If one compares the results between the studies using Lucentis at 24 months:
- MARINA: Mean VA improved by 7.2 letters, with a mean 24 injections
- ANCHOR: Mean VA improved by 11.1 letters, with a mean 24 injections
- PrONTO: Mean VA improved by 11.1 letters, with a mean 9.9 injections.

This suggests that OCT-guided treatment produces visual outcomes that are on par with monthly dosing.

Comparative ranibizumab and bevacizumab trials

The CATT and IVAN studies are 2 large trials that have compared the efficacy of Lucentis® (ranibizumab) and Avastin® (bevacizumab) intraocular injection, as well as continuous versus variable dosing regimes.

In the CATT trial, patients were randomized into 4 groups to receive either Lucentis or Avastin, with either a monthly or as needed administration (PRN) (without a 3 month loading dose). After 1 year the patients receiving monthly eye injections were re-randomized to continue receiving monthly injection, or switch to as needed. At 2 years there was no significant difference in letters gained between the Lucentis and Avastin groups, however patients receiving monthly injections gained approximately 2.5 more letters than in the PRN group. In addition, patients who switched from monthly injection to as needed after year 1, lost more letters at year 2 than those who were on an as needed regimen throughout. Development of geographic atrophy (mostly extra-foveal) was greater with the monthly regimen. No differences in death rates or arteriothrombotic events were found between the 2 drugs.

In the IVAN trial, patients were randomized to receive monthly Lucentis or Avastin, and either a monthly regime or PRN—which involved a loading dose of 3 monthly injections, followed by a further course of 3 injections if re-activity was detected. No significant difference in visual gain was found between drugs or treatment regimen. Arteriothrombotic events or heart failure occurred more commonly in patients receiving Lucentis, but there was no difference in death rates between the 2 drugs.

Aflibercept (Eylea®)

Aflibercept (Eylea, and formerly known as VEGF Trap-Eye) is a soluble fusion protein consisting of two extracellular cytokine receptor domains and a human Fc region of IgG. It binds to all forms of VEGF-A, VEGF-B and to placental growth factor (PDGF). The binding ability of Eylea is greater than previous anti-VEGF agents, and has a greater half-life than Lucentis (48–83 days versus 30 days).

Comparative Eylea versus Lucentis trials

VIEW 1 and 2 are two large phase 3 trials where patients were randomized to either, monthly 0.5 mg Lucentis, monthly 0.5 mg or 2 mg Eylea, or 2 mg of Eylea after a loading dose of 3 monthly injections. All Eylea doses and treatment regimes were non-inferior to the Lucentis group, and NICE has approved Eylea for wet AMD at the dose of 2 mg monthly for the first 3 months, followed by 2 mg every 2 months.

Ophthalmology at a Glance, Second Edition. Jane Olver, Lorraine Cassidy, Gurjeet Jutley, and Laura Crawley. © 2014 Jane Olver, Lorraine Cassidy,

138 Gurjeet Jutley and Laura Crawley. Published 2014 by John Wiley & Sons, Ltd. Companion Website: www.ataglanceseries.com/ophthal

Index

Page numbers in *italics* denote figures, those in **bold** denote tables.

Acanthamoeba keratitis *40*, 41, *81*, 82, 85
accommodation 27, *28*, 29, *36*, 56
acephalgic migraine 54
acetazolamide **136**
achromatopsia 107
acne rosacea 78
actinic keratosis *see* solar keratosis
aflibercept 138
age-related macular degeneration *34*, 52, 53, 57, *106*, 107, 123
  and cataract 55
  dry *26*, 107–8
  risk factors *106*
  wet *106*, 107–8
AIDS *see* HIV/AIDS
albinism *128*
alkali burns 45
allergic conjunctivitis *38*, 39, *64*, 65, 80
allergic eye disease 21, 80
allergic granulomatosis **132**
alpha-agonists **136**
alternate cover test *60*
altitudinal field defects *130*, 131
amblyopia *60*, 61
amethocaine 37
Amsler chart *26*, 27
ANCHOR study 138
angiography
  fluorescein *104*, *105*, 111
  indocyanine green *104*, 105
anisocoria, physiological *124*
anophthalmia 63, 73
anterior chamber *32*, 33, 48
anterior chamber angle *32*
anterior ischaemic optic neuropathy *50*, 54
anterior segment 32–3, *32*
aphakia 31
apraclonidine **136**
aqueous humour *96*
Argyll-Robinson pupil *125*
astigmatism 29, 56
atopic keratoconjunctivitis *38*, 39
atropine 37
autofluorescence 105
automated field analyser *24*, 25
Azopt **136**

B cell lymphoma, intraocular 119
bacterial keratitis 82
band keratopathy 48
basal cell carcinoma *66*, 67
Behçet's disease **132**
Bell's phenomenon 65
benign intracranial hypertension *50*, 51
Best's disease *106*, 107
beta-blockers **136**
betaxolol **136**
bevacizumab 138
Bielchowsky's sign *128*, 129
bimatoprost **136**

binocular single vision 61
bitemporal hemianopia 25, *130*, 131
blepharitis 65, *78*, 79
blind spot 25
blindness **18**
  certification 19
  children 123
  corneal 123
  economic 19
  global incidence *122*
  services and support 19
blood pressure control 111
blood-retinal barrier *106*
blowout fracture *44*, 45, 47
blunt injuries 46–7, *46*
branch retinal artery occlusion 53, *112*
branch retinal vein occlusion 53, *114*, 115
BRAVO study 116
brimonidine **136**
brinzolamide **136**
Bruch's membrane *34*, *104*, 105, *106*, **135**
bullous keratopathy 84
buphthalmos *62*, 63
BVOS study 116

canal of Schlemm *32*, 42
canaliculi 70
canaloplasty 101
Candida endophthalmitis 118
capillary haemangioma *64*, 65, 76
capsulopalpebral fascia *32*
carbonic anhydrase inhibitors **136**
Cardiff Acuity Test *58*, 59
caruncle *14*, *32*, 68
cataract *44*, *45*, 55, 56, 123
  assessment 89–91, *89*
  congenital 63, *89*
  post-uveitis 48
  postoperative care 94–5, *94*, **94**
  surgery 91, 92–3, *92*
cavernous haemangioma 74
central retinal artery occlusion *14*, *34*, 52, 53, *112*, 113
central retinal vein occlusion *34*, 52, 53, *114*, 115
cerebrovascular accident 54
chalazion *see* Meibomian cyst
chemical injuries *44*, 45
chemosis *32*, 33, *46*
cherry red spot 52
children 64–5, *64*
  blindness 123
  hyphaema 33
  ptosis *14*, *64*, 65
  retinoblastoma 33, 63
  retinoscopy *28*, 29
  strabismus 60–1, *61*
  visual acuity 58–9, *58*
  visual impairment **18**
Chlamydia trachomatis 39, 63, *120*, 121
chlamydial conjunctivitis 39
choriocapillaris *34*, 49, *104*, **135**
chorioretinitis *117*

choroid 48, 52, 105
  anatomy 104–5, *104*
  HIV-related infections *117*
  rupture 45
choroidal haemangioma 76
choroidal melanoma *76*, 77
choroidal naevus *76*, 77
choroidal neovascularization *106*
cicatricial pemphigoid *78*, 79
cilia *14*, *32*, *68*
ciliary artery 52
ciliary body 48
  hypotony 48
  innervation *36*
ciliary muscle *36*
cilioretinal artery 113
circle of Haller and Zinn 52
circumciliary injection *38*, 48
clinical trials 138
  see also individual trials
coloboma *62*, 63
colour blindness 27
colour vision testing *26*, 27
commotio retinae *44*, 45, 47
computed tomography 46
cone-rod dystrophy *106*, 107
cones *34*, *104*, *106*, **135**
confocal scanning laser ophthalmoscope 105
confrontation testing *24*, 25
conjunctiva 33, 38–9, *38*, 42, *66*
  chemosis *32*
  colour 33
  haemorrhage *38*
  laceration 45
  melanoma 76
  squamous cell carcinoma 77
conjunctival fornix *66*
conjunctival-corneal intraepithelial neoplasia *81*, 83
conjunctivitis 38–9, *38*, **134**
  allergic *38*, 39, *64*, 65, 80
  chlamydial 39
  giant papillary 39
  infective 39
  viral *38*
consensual reflex 27
constrictor pupillae *36*
contact lenses 30–1, *30*
  complications 85
  cosmetic 85
  indications 31
  keratitis *40*, 41
  medical uses 84–5, *84*
  painted 84
  tight lens syndrome 84
  types of 31
cornea *14*, *32*, 33, 40–1, *40*, *42*, 48, 81–3, *81*
  abrasion *32*, *40*, 41, 45, *46*, 47, **134**
  clarity 82
  cloudy 39
  diseases of *see specific conditions*
  foreign body *40*, *44*, 45, *46*, 47
  hereditary dystrophies 82–3

Ophthalmology at a Glance, Second Edition. Jane Olver, Lorraine Cassidy, Gurjeet Jutley, and Laura Crawley. © 2014 Jane Olver, Lorraine Cassidy, Gurjeet Jutley and Laura Crawley. Published 2014 by John Wiley & Sons, Ltd. Companion Website: www.ataglanceseries.com/ophthal